Strabismus

Siddharth Agrawal
Editor

Strabismus

For every Ophthalmologist

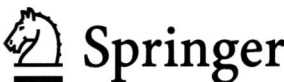 Springer

Editor
Siddharth Agrawal
Ophthalmology
King George's Medical University
Lucknow, Uttar Pradesh
India

ISBN 978-981-13-1125-3   ISBN 978-981-13-1126-0   (eBook)
https://doi.org/10.1007/978-981-13-1126-0

Library of Congress Control Number: 2018959277

This Springer imprint is published by Springer Nature, under the registered company Singapore Pte Ltd. The registered company address is: 152 Beach Road, #21-01/04 Gateway East, Singapore 189721, Singapore

Dedicated
to my father
Prof. G N Agrawal
who believed in academics
as the way forward for an intelligent mind
and
to my teacher
Prof. Vinita Singh
who introduced me
to strabismus and nurtured my interest in it.

Foreword

Strabismus is often regarded as a mystery not only by trainees but also by practising ophthalmologists. The practice of strabismus is an art as well as a science. The way we manage patients often reflects what we have learnt from a mentor and those who went before us.

Strabismus for every Ophthalmologist brings to the reader in a clear concise manner what we need to know to manage strabismus in a clinical setting.

Dr. Siddharth Agrawal has brought together a group of talented and experienced ophthalmologists from India and the Asia Pacific region to write an easy-to-read textbook covering all aspects of strabismus from basic to complex.

He has edited the book meticulously to ensure that each chapter follows the same format. The figures and diagrams are clear and reflect the vast clinical experience of the authors. Multiple choice questions towards the end of each chapter test the reader's understanding of each subject and will be invaluable to trainees in ophthalmology. Each chapter concludes with a very complete list of references.

This is not just another textbook on strabismus. It is a very readable manuscript and I regard it as a testament to the vast clinical experience of the authors.

Frank J. Martin
Clinical Professor, University of Sydney
Visiting Medical Officer, Sydney Children's Hospitals Network
Chairman, Children's Medical Research Institute Sydney
Director, Sydney Ophthalmic Specialists
Sydney, NSW, Australia

Acknowledgements

This book was conceptualised during a workshop jointly organised by Dr. Naren Aggarwal, Associate Editorial Director, Clinical Medicine, Springer, and Prof. Apul Goel, Urology, King George's Medical University (KGMU), Lucknow, India, with the aim to simplify the rather complex topic of strabismus, for all ophthalmologists, specifically the postgraduate students.

Dr. Rajat M. Srivastava, Assistant Professor, Ophthalmology, KGMU, more a friend than a colleague has worked equally hard with me, going through the entire manuscript and suggesting improvements. Dr. Neha Singh, my Senior Resident, and Dr. Ankur Yadav, my Clinical Fellow, have been involved in nearly all the photographs, diagrams and tables. They are truly brilliant and have a bright future. Prof. Vinita Singh, the head of my department, provided the appropriate environment for this work.

I sincerely thank all the contributors who have trusted me with their work. I hope they are as proud of this book as I am. Patients and students are central to all my clinical and academic work. They are the motivating force behind anything constructive that I do.

A happy environment at home is essential for any kind of growth, and I thank my family specially my talented wife Neha, for the same.

Siddharth Agrawal
April, 2018

Contents

Contributors

Siddharth Agrawal Department of Ophthalmology, King George's Medical University, Lucknow, India

Joyce Chan Hong Kong Eye Hospital, Kowloon, Hong Kong

Rolli Khurana Dr. Shroff's Charity Eye Hospital, Delhi, India

Carol P. S. Lam Hong Kong Eye Hospital, Kowloon, Hong Kong

Winnie W. Y. Lau Hong Kong Eye Hospital, Kowloon, Hong Kong

Swati Phuljhele Dr. Rajendra Prasad Centre for Ophthalmic Sciences, All India Institute of Medical Sciences (AIIMS), New Delhi, India

Manu Saini Dr. Rajendra Prasad Centre for Ophthalmic Sciences, All India Institute of Medical Sciences (AIIMS), New Delhi, India

Rohit Saxena Dr. Rajendra Prasad Centre for Ophthalmic Sciences, All India Institute of Medical Sciences (AIIMS), New Delhi, India

Pradeep Sharma Dr. Rajendra Prasad Centre for Ophthalmic Sciences, All India Institute of Medical Sciences (AIIMS), New Delhi, India

Neha Singh Department of Ophthalmology, King George's Medical University, Lucknow, India

Priyanka Singh Aravind Eye Hospital, Madurai, India

Vinita Singh Department of Ophthalmology, King George's Medical University, Lucknow, India

Rajat M. Srivastava Department of Ophthalmology, King George's Medical University, Lucknow, India

Chong-Bin Tsai Department of Ophthalmology, Chiayi Christian Hospital, Chiayi City, Taiwan

Department of Hospital and Health Care Administration, Chia Nan University of Pharmacy and Science, Chiayi, Taiwan

Ankur Yadav Department of Ophthalmology, King George's Medical University, Lucknow, India

Jason C. S. Yam Hong Kong Eye Hospital, Kowloon City, Hong Kong

Department of Ophthalmology and Visual Sciences, The Chinese University of Hong Kong, Shatin, Hong Kong

Basics of Understanding Strabismus

Vinita Singh, Siddharth Agrawal, Neha Singh,
and Ankur Yadav

1.1 Introduction

It is often perplexing to see a patient with deviated eyes and random-appearing eye movements. 'The strabismus puzzle' can be a daunting task for anyone in the absence of lucid understanding of the motor and sensory mechanisms that govern ocular alignment and movement.

1.2 What Is Strabismus?

Strabismus may be defined as the *inability of the two eyes to simultaneously direct their foveae at a common object of regard, occasionally or always.*

In slightly technical terms, it is the inability of both the eyes to align their visual axes to common object of regard, visual axis being the line joining the fovea of the eye to the fixation point [1].

1.3 How Do the Eyes Remain Aligned?

Both the eyes, the extraocular muscles and the nervous system function together as a sensorimotor unit to keep the eyes aligned. An intact sensory system enables us to binocularly perceive our surroundings in depth (i.e. in third dimension). The motor system moves the eyes to bring the object of attention onto the fovea and aligns both the eyes to enable binocular single vision. Both the systems work in unison and are mutually reinforcing for each other. A defect in either of them may result in strabismus.

V. Singh · S. Agrawal (✉) · N. Singh · A. Yadav
Department of Ophthalmology, King George's Medical University, Lucknow, India

© Springer Nature Singapore Pte Ltd. 2019
S. Agrawal (ed.), *Strabismus*, https://doi.org/10.1007/978-981-13-1126-0_1

1.4   Understanding the Motor Mechanisms

These comprise of a neuromuscular complex of extraocular muscles and cranial nerves which synchronise various ocular movements and maintain ocular alignment. There are six extraocular muscles attached to the globe, which cause its movement in various directions. The rotation of the globe occurs along the X (up and down), Y (torsion) and Z (left and right) axes (of Fick). These axes intersect at an imaginary coronal plane of Listing (Fig. 1.1).

1.4.1   Extraocular Muscles

Four recti (superior, inferior, medial, lateral) muscles and two oblique (superior, inferior) muscles comprise the extraocular muscles. All the four recti muscles originate from the annulus of Zinn and insert anterior to the equator of the eye at varying distances from the limbus, depicting a spiral pattern (spiral of Tillaux). Since their insertions lie anteriorly, they primarily tug at the anterior pole of the eye (Fig. 1.2).

The superior and the inferior recti are known as the 'vertical recti', and they move the eye in vertical plane. Similarly, the medial and the lateral recti are known as the 'horizontal recti', and they move the eye in horizontal plane. All the recti

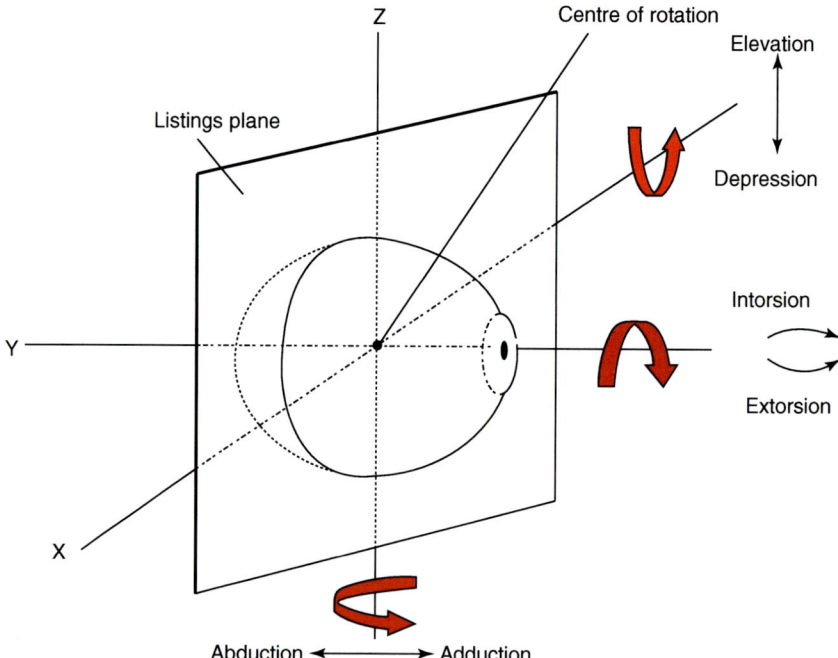

Fig. 1.1 Fick axes and Listing plane. X axis is nasal to temporal (elevation and depression occur on it), Y axis is anterior to posterior (intorsion and extorsion occur on it), Z axis is superior to inferior (abduction and adduction occur on it). Note that the X and Y axes lie in the horizontal plane

muscles are innervated by the oculomotor nerve except for the lateral rectus, which is innervated by the abducens nerve.

The oblique muscles are so named as they lie oblique to the visual axis making an angle of about 51°. The superior oblique originates superomedial to the optic foramen, above the annulus of Zinn. The muscle traverses anteriorly in the supero-medial orbit before passing through the trochlea, changing its direction posterolaterally to get inserted on the supero-posterior-temporal aspect of the eye. The inferior oblique has a rather simpler course. It originates in the anterior orbit from a depression near the lacrimal fossa and inserts on the infero-posterior-temporal aspect of the eye. Since the insertion of both the oblique muscles lies posterior to the equator of the eye, they primarily tug at the posterior pole moving the anterior pole in the opposite directions (Fig. 1.3). The superior oblique is innervated by the trochlear nerve, and the inferior oblique is innervated by the oculomotor nerve.

Fig. 1.2 The insertion of recti depicting the spiral of Tillaux. The insertion distances from the limbus in millimetres are maximum values and may vary amongst individuals

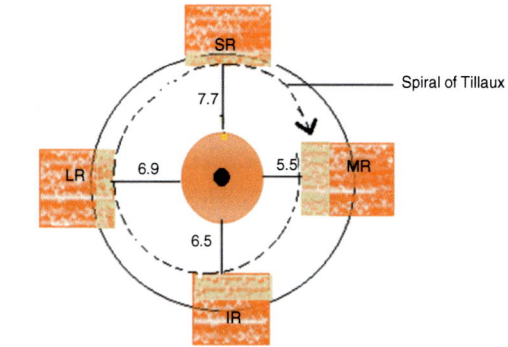

Fig. 1.3 Insertion of the superior oblique and the angle between muscle plane (MA) and visual axis (VA)

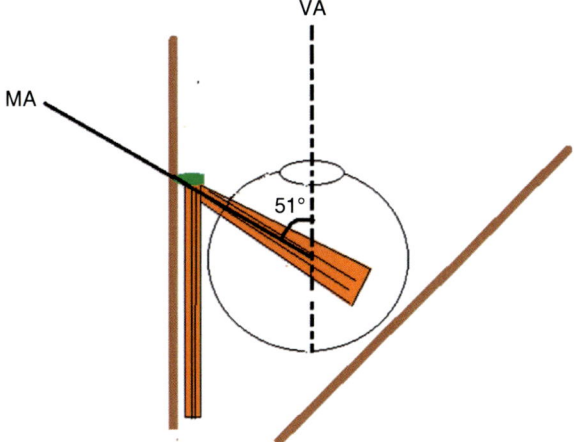

1.4.2 Ocular Movements

It is essential to understand that all ocular movements are rotatory movements around the Fick's axes (explained earlier). A complex and synchronised neuromuscular interaction between extraocular muscles is responsible for precise ocular movements. All ocular movements, when described uniocularly, are termed as 'ductions', whereas binocularly are termed 'versions' (conjugate movements) and 'vergence' (disconjugate movements). Functional motility is demonstrated by versions and is hence more important [2]. Ductions demonstrate the maximum movement possible with the strongest innervational impulse. A limited duction is usually due to a significant muscle palsy or mechanical restriction. Comparison between the two eyes is essential for any useful clinical observation.

1.4.2.1 Uniocular Movements: Ductions

When the globe moves in the horizontal plane, its nasal movement is called *adduction*, and temporal movement is called *abduction*. In the vertical plane, upward movement is called *elevation* and downward movement is *depression*. These four movements are called the cardinal movements of the eye. Nasal movement of the 12 o'clock limbus along the anteroposterior axis is called *intorsion*, and its temporal movement is called *extorsion*. These movements are elicited by making a person follow a fixation target uniocularly. Table 1.1 summarises the movements of the extraocular muscles in primary position (Fig. 1.4).

1.4.2.2 Binocular Movements: Versions

Versions are binocular conjugate movements, i.e. both eyes look in the same direction. In the horizontal plane when *both* the eyes look towards the right, the movement is called *dextroversion*, and the movement towards left is called

Table 1.1 Action of extraocular muscles in primary position (when looking straight ahead with the body and head erect)

	Primary action	Secondary action	Tertiary action
Medial rectus	Adduction		
Lateral rectus	Abduction		
Superior rectus	Elevation	Intorsion	Adduction
Inferior rectus	Depression	Extorsion	Adduction
Superior oblique	Intorsion	Depression	Abduction
Inferior oblique	Extorsion	Elevation	Abduction

Ocular rotation is determined by the movement of the 12 o'clock point on the limbus along the anteroposterior axis. Inward (towards nose) movement is intorsion (or incycloduction), and the outward movement is extorsion (or excycloduction)

The secondary actions of the vertical recti become maximal in abduction and of obliques in adduction. In fact, the inferior oblique is pure elevator and superior oblique pure depressor in extreme adduction

To memorise it should be noticed that the superior muscles are intorters and inferior muscles are extorters. The vertical recti are adductors. The obliques are abductors although their maximal vertical action is in adduction

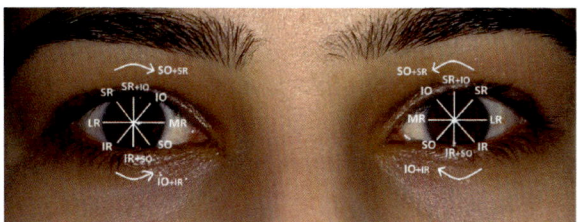

Fig. 1.4 Photograph shows the representation of the ocular motility, i.e. the muscles responsible for various movements. *IO* inferior oblique, *IR* inferior rectus, *LR* lateral rectus, *IR* inferior rectus, *SO* superior oblique, *MR* medial rectus

levoversion. Similarly, upward binocular movement is called *elevation* (or up gaze), and downward movement is *depression* (or down gaze). Binocular rotation along the anteroposterior axis of the upper limbus to the right is called *dextrocycloversion* and to the left is called *levocycloversion*. Movement to right and up is called dextroelevation. Similarly, the gazes dextrodepression, levoelevation and levodepression are named. Levoversion, levoelevation, levodepression, dextroversion, dextroelevation and dextrodepression are collectively called six cardinal gazes.

1.4.2.3 Binocular Movements: Vergences

Vergences are disconjugate ocular movements, i.e. both eyes look in different directions. These are complex binocular movements that occur to maintain fusion. Unlike versions, both eyes together move nasally (*convergence*) or temporally (*divergence*) and are thus also termed as disjunctive movements [3]. Besides horizontal vergences, vertical and cyclofusional movements also occur, but they are of limited clinical importance for the general ophthalmologist.

These movements represent the motor aspect of fusion and have an amplitude which is greatest for convergence. All vergences occur as a reflex; however, convergence is the only vergence movement that may also be voluntary. Reflex convergence has four components: (1) tonic (due to inherent tone of medial recti), (2) proximal (induced by psychological awareness of an object in proximity), (3) fusional (induced by bitemporal retinal image disparity) and (4) accommodative (induced as a part of synkinetic near reflex).

It is believed that the stimulus for motor fusion arises in the retinal periphery and it enables fusion within a range even when retinal disparity occurs outside the Panum's area (discussed later).

1.4.3 Agonist/Antagonist and Synergist/Yoke Muscles

A muscle which moves the eye in a particular direction is called an *agonist*, and the muscle which moves the globe in opposite direction is called its *antagonist*. For example, the lateral rectus abducts the eye, and the medial rectus adducts it making these two muscles antagonists of each other. Two muscles in the same eye moving it in same direction are called *synergists*. For example, both the inferior oblique and superior rectus elevate the eye and are synergists for this movement.

When binocular movements are considered, one muscle in each eye is responsible for a particular gaze, like the right medial rectus and left lateral rectus that contract during levoversion. These pairs of muscles are called the *yoke* muscles.

1.4.4   Neuromotor Complex

As now evident from the above discussion, ocular movements occur not merely by individual muscles rotating the eyes but are a complex and precise interaction between extraocular muscles of the eyes. The neuromotor complex governing ocular movements is best explained by the following laws of innervations:

'Hering's law of equal innervation': The law states that *equal* innervational impulses (to contract or relax) are sent to the *corresponding* (*yoke*) muscles of each eye whenever an eye movement occurs [5].

'Sherrington's law of reciprocal innervation': The law states that when a muscle receives an impulse to contract, an *equivalent inhibitory* impulse is sent to *its antagonist* which relaxes and lengthens it [6].

To understand these laws, let us take an example where the right eye follows an object and moves outwards (abducts). To execute this movement, the brain sends an impulse to contract to the right lateral rectus (RLR). An equal impulse to contract is also sent to the left medial rectus (yoke muscle of RLR). This is in accordance with Hering's law. As RLR receives the impulse to contract, an equivalent inhibitory impulse to relax is sent out to the right medial rectus (antagonist of RLR). This explains the Sherrington's law.

There are *six cardinal gazes* which are important clinically, as they are used to determine the paralysed and the overacting muscles. The following photograph (Fig. 1.5) depicts these gazes and the pair of yoke muscles responsible for them. These six gazes, the primary position, direct elevation and depression form the *nine diagnostic gazes* for examination of versions.

1.5   Understanding the Sensory Mechanisms

The sensory mechanisms are the driving force of the motor mechanisms. These reinforce the motor mechanisms to maintain ocular alignment and precisely coordinate ocular movements. The components of sensory mechanisms include the following:

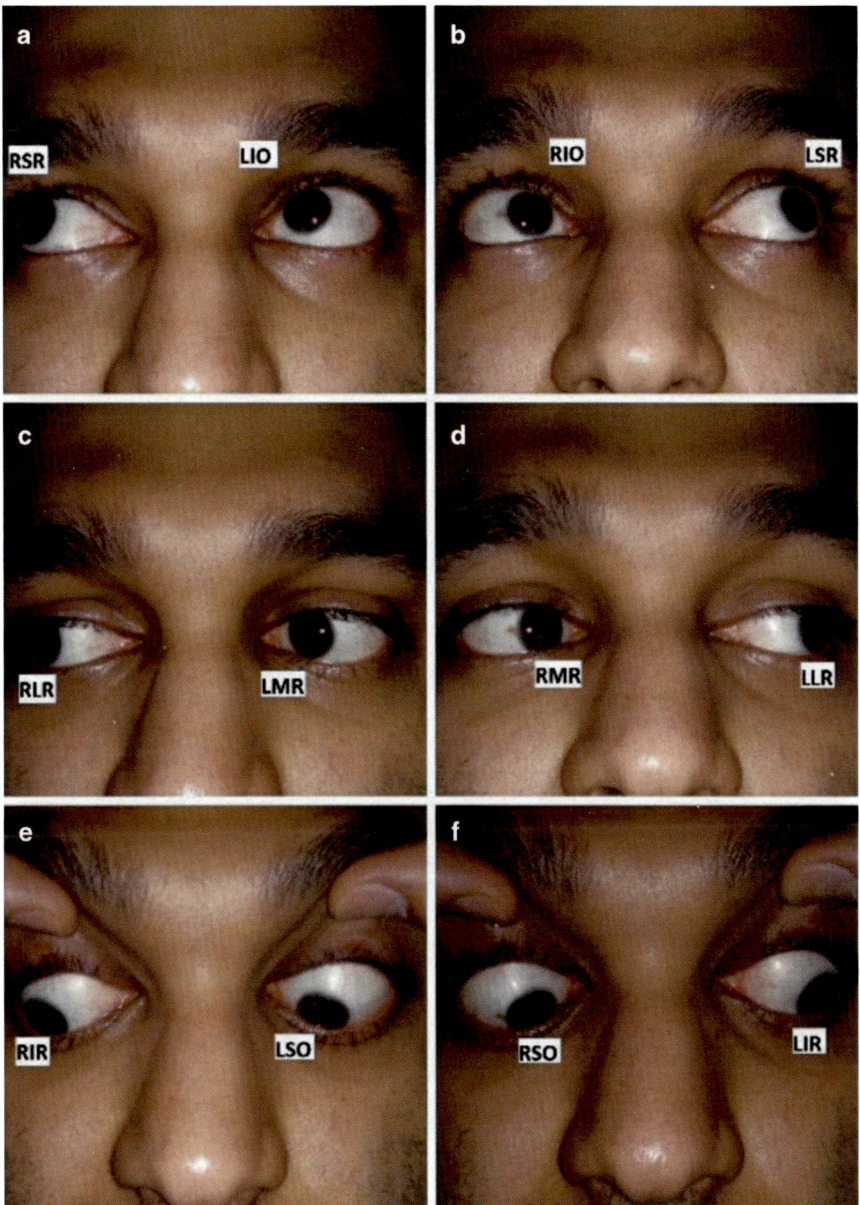

Fig. 1.5 Photograph showing six cardinal gazes and yoke muscles acting in them. (**a**) dextroeleva-tion, (**b**) levoelevation, (**c**) dextroversion, (**d**) levoversion, (**e**) dextrodepression, (**f**) levodepression. *LIO* left inferior oblique, *LIR* left inferior rectus, *LLR* left lateral rectus, *LIR* left inferior rectus, *LSO* left superior oblique, *LMR* left medial rectus, *RIO* right inferior oblique, *RMR* right medial rectus, *RSO* right superior oblique, *RIR* right inferior rectus, *RLR* right lateral rectus, *RSR* right superior rectus

1.5.1   Binocular Single Vision (BSV)

Binocular single vision (BSV) involves simultaneous contribution of both eyes to perceive a single image of the object of regard. It is the single most important sensory mechanism driving motor ocular alignment.

1.5.2   Corresponding Retinal Points and Horopter

Binocular single vision is the product of precise motor and sensory interaction between eyes. The points on the retina of one eye correspond with retinal points of the other eye, i.e. stimulation of these two points causes a subjective perception that the stimulating target shares the same spatial character (direction and orientation) in space around us. Both the foveae (in the presence of normal retinal correspondence) are corresponding points and share the primary visual direction. Points on the nasal retina of one eye correspond with points on the temporal retina of the other eye. Image of an object falling on the corresponding retinal points is perceived as single and if falling on non-corresponding (or *disparate*) retinal points is perceived as double (*diplopia*) which provides the feedback to correct any motor cause. Each retinal point has a corresponding spatial coordinate (locus). A horopter is an imaginary line joining the spatial loci of all the corresponding retinal points in space around us. It should be understood that the horopter would change depending on the fixation point which would be unique and centred on that point.

1.5.3   Panum's Area of Binocular Single Vision

Panum's area is a zone in front and behind the horopter, in which slightly non-corresponding retinal points are stimulated but are seen as single. The stimulation of nearby non-corresponding points causes perception of binocular depth or *stereopsis*. This area is narrow near the fixation and becomes broader towards the periphery (Fig. 1.6). Objects outside the Panum's area fall on distant non-corresponding retinal points and are perceived as double. This forms the basis of physiological diplopia. Ocular motor alignment is necessary for binocular single vision and stereopsis to develop.

1.5.4   Fusion

Unification of visual images from the two eyes to be perceived as one in the cerebral cortex is termed as fusion. For fusion to occur, the retinal images must be of similar size, shape and clarity. More dissimilarity is tolerated in the periphery (peripheral fusion) compared to areas near the fovea (central fusion), before diplopia occurs. Two separate components of fusion are often discussed although they work in unison.

Sensory fusion is contributed by the corresponding (or nearby non-corresponding) retinal points, visual pathways and cortex. Motor fusion is a vergence movement (as

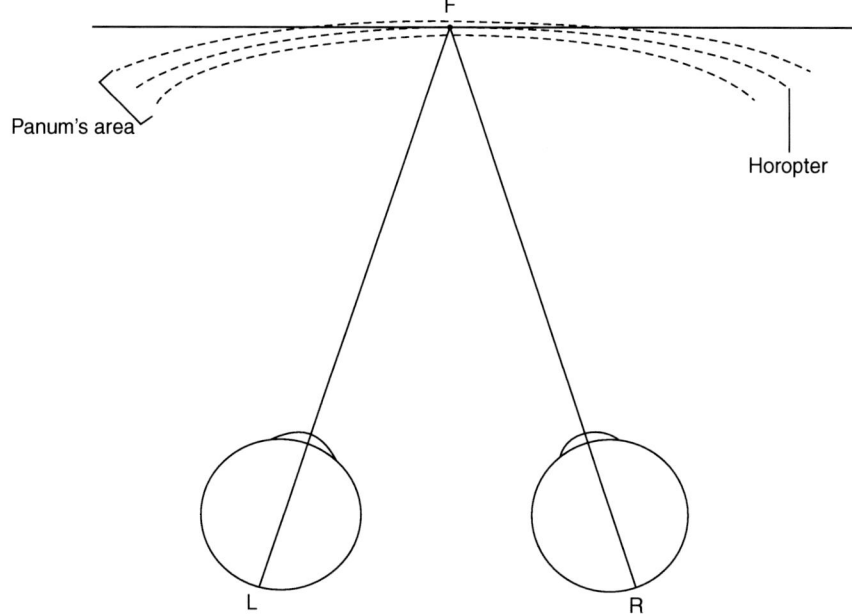

Fig. 1.6 The horopter and Panum's fusional area. FL and FR represent the visual axes of the left and right eye, respectively. The Panum's fusional area is narrower near fixation and broader towards the periphery

detailed earlier) enabling similar retinal images to be maintained on corresponding retinal points. Sensory fusion occurs for disparity within the Panum's area, and motor fusional movements (e.g. fusional convergence) occur when disparity exceeds this area [3]. When fusional range is overwhelmed, binocular single vision would not be possible.

1.5.5   Stereopsis

The horizontal separation of eyes causes images of a single object of regard falling on both the foveae to be slightly dissimilar as each eye views the same object from a slightly different angle (equal to angle between the two visual axes). Sensory fusion of these two dissimilar images results in three-dimensional perception of the object, called stereopsis. Normal range of stereopsis in young individuals is between 25 and 40 s of arc on Randot circle test (Stereo Optical Co., Inc., Chicago, IL, USA) [4].

In normal conditions, monocular clues besides stereopsis also contribute to perception of depth. These clues include overlap of objects, relative size of objects, highlights and shadows, motion parallax and perspective. The major role in depth perception at near is played by stereopsis and at distance by monocular clues.

1.6   Normal Ocular Alignment

Orthophoria is perfect ocular alignment without any stimulus for fusion. This usually does not occur, and a certain amount of heterophoria is commoner in normal population [5].

Orthotropia is a better term implying a negative cover test (on covering either eye) in the absence of amblyopia. Orthotropia is present in normal individuals and is the desirable end stage of strabismus treatment.

Having understood the mechanisms involved in maintaining ocular alignment and precise ocular movements, we can now understand the aberrations in motor and sensory mechanisms in strabismus.

1.7   Abnormalities in Ocular Alignment

Heterophoria or latent strabismus is deviation of the eyes in the absence of stimulus for fusion. The deviation may be inwards (esophoria) or outwards (exophoria). This condition is usually physiological with the eyes remaining aligned in normal conditions with both eyes open. However, when the fusional reflex becomes insufficient to overcome this latent deviation, the individual may develop symptoms like diplopia or asthenopia.

Heterotropia or manifest strabismus occurs when the visual axes of both the eyes are misaligned (or do not intersect at the fixation point). Simply put, it is the inability of the eyes to fixate simultaneously at the object of regard.

Heterotropia may be esotropia or exotropia depending on whether the visual axes (and the eyes) converge or diverge. It may also be hypertropia or hypotropia depending on whether the non-fixating eye is above or below the fixating eye. For example, in left hypertropia, the right eye is fixating and the left eye is higher to it. Similarly cyclotropia refers to clockwise and counterclockwise misalignment around the sagittal axis.

The deviation may be present at all the times (*constant*) or be controlled by fusion under certain conditions (*intermittent*). At the same time, the deviation may be greater or lesser at certain times, when it is called *variable*.

1.8   Abnormalities in Sensory Mechanisms

In the presence of heterotropia, corresponding retinal elements of the eyes are unable to focus at the same object. This may lead to the following sensory aberrations.

Confusion occurs when different objects project on the fovea of each eye. The foveae are physiologically unable to simultaneously perceive two dissimilar objects which to the patient may either appear to rapidly alternate (*retinal rivalry*) or appear superimposed [6] (Fig. 1.7). Clinically this is seldom observed [6].

Diplopia or double vision is usually observed after acquired heterotropia. It occurs as the image of the same object falls on the fovea of one eye and a non-foveal point outside the Panum's area of the other eye. Diplopia is termed as uncrossed and crossed depending on whether the image projected from the deviated eye falls on the same side or on the opposite side (Fig. 1.8). The foveal image being clearer, the individual may learn to *suppress* the non-foveal image of the non-fixating eye, as discussed in the later. The ability to suppress is greater in young children.

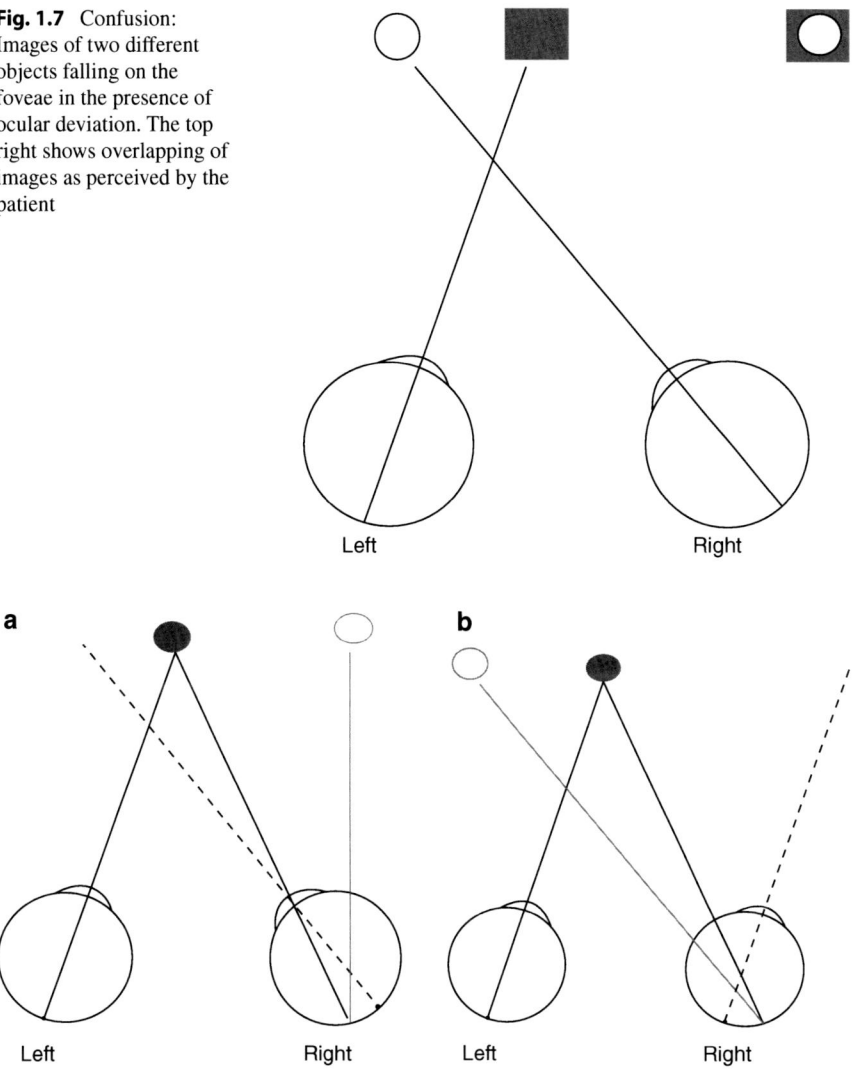

Fig. 1.7 Confusion: Images of two different objects falling on the foveae in the presence of ocular deviation. The top right shows overlapping of images as perceived by the patient

Fig. 1.8 Diplopia. (**a**) Uncrossed (homonymous) diplopia in esotropia. The solid circle represents the object whose image forms on the fovea of the left eye (LE) and on the nasal retina of the deviated right eye (RE). The dotted line represents the projection of fovea of RE, and the hollow circle represents the false (second) image projected by the RE. (**b**) Crossed (heteronymous) diplopia in exotropia (XT). The image of the object falls on the temporal retina of RE which is projected nasally. Hence, when the image of the right eye forms on the right, the diplopia is termed as uncrossed, and when it forms on the left, it is termed as crossed

1.9 Motor Adaptations in Strabismus

In the presence of strabismus, motor adaptations provide an opportunity to enjoy binocular single vision. Motor adaptation in strabismus may occur in the form of excessive vergence to attain fusion or by adopting anomalous head posture (AHP) also called compensatory head posture (CHP). This is a feature of incomitant strabismus (discussed later) with the patient adopting a head posture that minimises diplopia and maximises the field of binocular single vision. The AHP has three components, (a) face turn, (b) head tilt and (c) chin elevation or depression (Fig. 1.9).

An interesting phenomenon of Swann's blind spot mechanism may be seen in small-angle constant esotropia where the image in the deviated eye falls over the optic disc (blind spot) [7]. Diplopia is thus avoided without causing suppression.

1.10 Sensory Adaptations in Strabismus

In the presence of strabismus, to avoid confusion and diplopia, the visual system adopts one of the following mechanisms. These mechanisms usually develop in the visually immature system, i.e. in children lesser than 6–8 years of age.

1.10.1 Suppression

Suppression is active central inhibition of the image from one eye when both eyes are open. It should be noted that suppression occurs during conditions of binocular viewing only as against amblyopia which persists even when the better eye is closed [8].

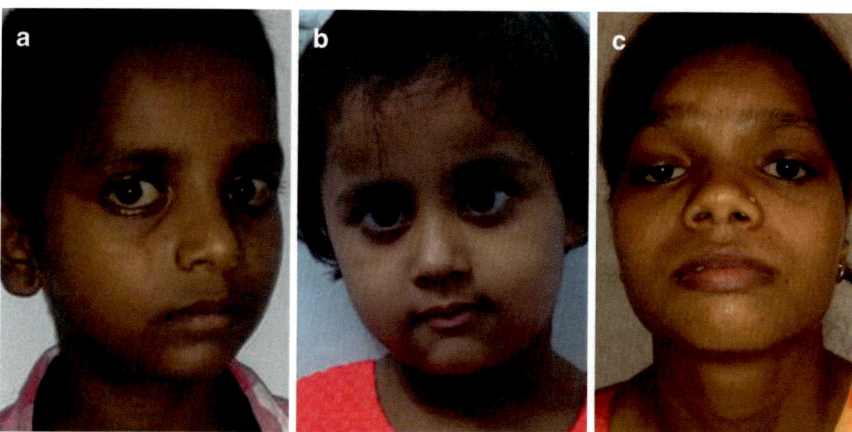

Fig. 1.9 Three components of anomalous head posture (AHP) have been shown: (**a**) face turn, (**b**) head tilt and (**c**) chin elevation

Suppression can be *central or peripheral* depending on whether the image from the fovea of deviating eye is suppressed to avoid confusion or that from the peripheral retina is suppressed to avoid diplopia. It may also be *monocular or alternating* depending on whether the same eye is always suppressing or both the eyes are taking turns as is observed in alternating exotropia. Monocular suppression may eventually lead to amblyopia. Suppression may also be classified as *facultative or constant* depending on whether it is present only when the eyes are deviated or is also present when the eyes are aligned. Facultative suppression is seen in intermittent exotropia which allows the patients to avoid diplopia when the eyes are squinting and enjoy stereopsis when they are aligned.

1.10.2 Abnormal Retinal Correspondence

In the presence of long-standing, early-onset, small-angle, constant heterotropia (frequently esotropia [9]), a non-foveal point of the deviated eye develops correspondence with the fovea of the fixating eye. This is called abnormal retinal correspondence (ARC) and is a superior functional state compared to suppression as it allows subnormal levels of binocular vision in the presence of heterotropia [10].

ARC is usually diagnosed after childhood, and as such its treatment is not indicated as it may result in intractable diplopia [11].

Another sensory adaptation is *eccentric fixation* which is usually a monocular phenomenon (unlike ARC which occurs during binocular viewing). In this the eye utilises a portion of the retina other than the fovea for fixation. It frequently occurs in strabismic amblyopia and is associated with poor visual acuity [12].

1.11 Classification of Strabismus

Understanding the presentation of strabismus would be a good beginning to solving the puzzle. Strabismus can be broadly classified into two major forms, *comitant* and *incomitant*. Strabismus is called comitant (also called concomitant) when for a particular fixation distance the deviation is same in all directions of gaze. It is incomitant when the deviation varies in different gazes or with the eye used for fixation. Incomitant strabismus is usually *paralytic* (due to palsy of the third, fourth or sixth cranial nerve) or *restrictive* (due to involvement of extraocular ocular muscles or their surrounding soft tissue).

Primary deviation is the deviation when the normal eye is fixating, and *secondary deviation* is the deviation when the paretic or the restricted eye is fixating (Fig. 1.10). Secondary deviations are larger.

Differences between comitant and incomitant strabismus are listed in Table 1.2.

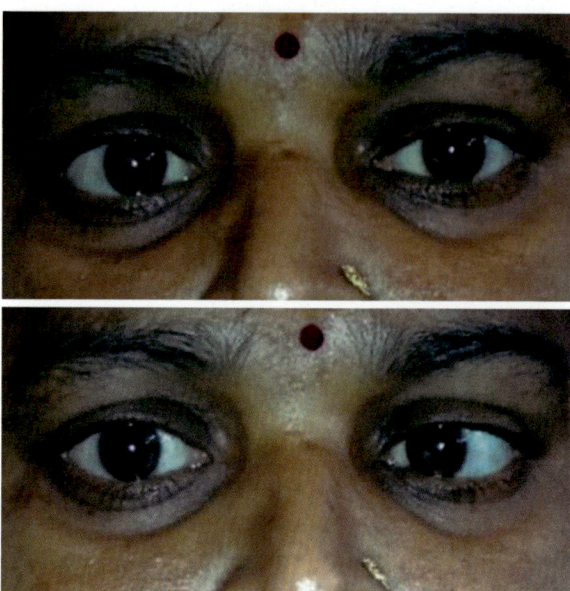

Fig. 1.10 Primary and secondary deviations in right lateral rectus paresis. In the upper photograph, the left (nonparetic) eye is fixating, and the esotropia in the right (paretic) eye is the *primary deviation*. In the lower photograph, the right eye is fixating, and the larger deviation in the nonparetic (left) eye is the *secondary deviation*

Table 1.2 Differences between comitant and incomitant strabismus

	Comitant	Incomitant
Symptoms		
Onset	Insidious	Sudden usually following trauma, viral illness, neurosurgery, poor glycaemic control or hypertension
Duration	Usually since childhood	Usually recent
Diplopia	No	Yes
Signs		
Head posture (motor adaptation)	No	Yes
Motility limitation	No	Yes
Secondary deviation > primary deviation	No	Yes
Sensory adaptations	Yes	No

1.12 Few Other Important Concepts

The *visual axis* connects the fovea with the point of fixation [1]. In normal conditions, the visual axes of two eyes intersect at the point of fixation, and the motor and sensory components discussed above enable binocular single vision.

The *pupillary axis* (or the anatomical axis) is the line passing through the centre of the pupil and perpendicular to the cornea. When extended posteriorly, it touches the posterior pole of the globe slightly nasal and inferior to the fovea (Fig. 1.11). This implies that when an eye would fixate on a penlight, the reflection from the cornea would appear slightly nasal to the centre (Fig. 1.12). This is termed positive angle kappa and is physiological. *Angle kappa* is the angle formed at the intersection of visual and pupillary axes and is usually about 5°. It makes an exotropia appear larger and may mask an esotropia [13].

1.13 Summary

- Normal ocular alignment and motility are a result of complex interaction between the motor and sensory mechanisms of the eye.
- Motor mechanisms comprise of the extraocular muscles and cranial nerves innervating them.
- Binocular single vision and fusion are important sensory mechanisms maintaining ocular alignment.
- Strabismus is relative misalignment of visual axes of eyes occurring as a consequence of altered sensory and motor mechanisms.

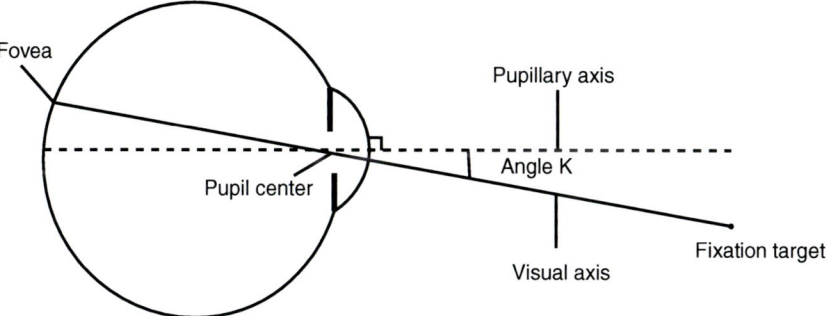

Fig. 1.11 Angle kappa is formed between pupillary axis and visual axis at the centre of the pupil

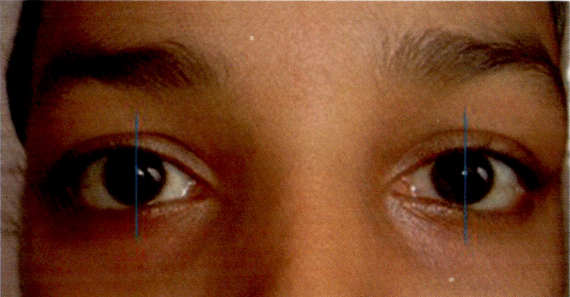

Fig. 1.12 The lines represent the plane of pupillary axis and divide the pupils into two equal halves. The corneal light reflexes fall nasally (more prominent on the right side) attributed to positive angle kappa. The eyes are straight on cover test

- Compensatory head posture, blind spot mechanism and excessive convergence are motor adaptations seen in strabismus. Suppression, amblyopia, eccentric fixation and abnormal retinal correspondence are some of the sensory adaptations.
- Strabismus is called comitant when the angle of deviation remains equal in all the gazes. When the angle of deviation varies with gaze, it is termed incomitant.
- In paralytic strabismus, deviation observed with the normal eye and paralytic eye fixating is termed as primary and secondary deviation, respectively. Secondary deviation is larger than primary deviation.

1.14 Multiple Choice Questions

1. Which of the following statements is correct?
    (a) The superior rectus is inserted closest to the limbus amongst the recti muscles.
    (b) Strabismus can occur in a single-eyed person.
    (c) The oblique muscles are inserted on the sclera posterior to the equator medial to the vertical recti.
    (d) The visual axis is the line joining the fovea of the eye to the fixation point.

Answer: (d) The medial rectus inserts closest to the limbus. Strabismus is misalignment of the visual axes of the two eyes relative to each other which cannot occur in a single-eyed person. The obliques are inserted posterior to the equator, lateral to the insertion of the vertical recti.

2. Ductions are the uniocular eye movements and versions are the binocular movements. Which of the following statements is true regarding them?
    (a) The inferior oblique causes extorsion, elevation and abduction.
    (b) The superior oblique causes depression when the eye is abducted.
    (c) Tertiary action of the vertical recti is abduction.
    (d) Ductions may not be evaluated if the versions are limited.

Answer: (a) The superior oblique causes depression in adduction. Adduction is the tertiary action of the vertical recti. Ductions should always be evaluated when the versions are found to be limited.

3. Fusion is unification of the images from the two eyes in the cerebral cortex. All of the following conditions are essential for fusion to occur *except*:
    (a) The images should be of similar size, shape and clarity.
    (b) The image of the object must fall on the corresponding retinal points in the two eyes.
    (c) Absence of strabismus.
    (d) Intact visual pathways.

Answer: (c) Fusion can occur in the presence of strabismus with the patient adopting a compensatory (or anomalous) head posture, by use of prisms, and in the presence of abnormal retinal correspondence (ARC).

4. Which of the following is true regarding differentiation between concomitant and incomitant strabismus?
   (a) Primary deviation is larger than the secondary in incomitant deviations.
   (b) Diplopia is a feature of recent-onset incomitant deviations.
   (c) Sensory adaptations occur in incomitant deviations.
   (d) Motor adaptations occur in comitant deviations.

Answer: (b) Secondary deviation is larger than the primary in incomitant strabismus. Sensory adaptations like suppression occur commonly in comitant strabismus. Motor adaptations like anomalous head posture are a feature of incomitant deviations.

References

1. Lancaster WB. Refraction correlated with optics and physiological optics and motility limited to heterophoria. Springfield, IL: Charles C Thomas; 1952. p. 102.
2. Bielschowsky A. Lectures on motor anomalies. Hannover, NH: Dartmouth College Publications; 1943/1956.
3. von Noorden GK, Campos EC. Chapter 4: Physiology of ocular movements. In: Binocular vision and ocular motility. 6th ed. St. Louis: Mosby; 2002. p. 71–6.
4. Lee SY, Koo NK. Change of stereoacuity with aging in normal eyes. Korean J Ophthalmol. 2005;19(2):136–9.
5. Bielschowsky A. Uber die ruhelage der Augen, vol 66. Bericht 39. Versammlung ophthalmologische Gesellschaft, Heidelberg. Wiesbaden, JF Bergmann, p. 67 ff; 1913.
6. Cantor LB, Rapuano CJ, Cioffi GA. Chapter 6: Sensory physiology and pathology. In: Basic and clinical science course 2015–16, Section 6. San Francisco, CA: American Academy of Ophthalmology. p. 53–64.
7. Swan KG. The blindspot syndrome. Arch Ophthalmol. 1948;40(4):371–88.
8. von Noorden GK, Campos EC. Chapter 13: Examination of patient III. In: Binocular vision and ocular motility. 6th ed. St. Louis: Mosby; 2002. p. 211–45.
9. De Belsunce S, Sireteanu R. The time course of interocular suppression in normal and amblyopic subjects. Invest Ophthalmol Vis Sci. 1991;32:2645.
10. Herzau V. How useful is anomalous correspondence? Eye. 1996;10:266.
11. Quere MA, Lavenant G, Pechereau A, et al. Les diplopies incoercibles post-therapeutiques. J Fr Orthopt. 1993;25:191.
12. von Noorden GK. Pathophysiology of amblyopia: diagnostic and therapeutic principles of pleoptics. Am Orthopt J. 1960;10:7.
13. Von Noorden GK, Campos EC. Chapter 12: Examination of the patient II. In: Binocular vision and ocular motility. 6th ed. St. Louis: Mosby; 2002. p. 169–74.

Clinical Evaluation of Strabismus

2

Siddharth Agrawal, Ankur Yadav, and Neha Singh

2.1 Introduction

It is not uncommon in an ophthalmologist's office to have an anxious couple with the complaint of their child squinting occasionally. Confirming the presence or absence of deviation requires patience and a systematic approach. Even if obvious, the ophthalmologist should not comment on the deviation till completion of examination.

2.2 History Taking

In a patient with suspicion of strabismus, a detailed history including the onset, duration, intermittency, aggravating or relieving factors, associated ocular and systemic complaints, should be elicited. Specific importance to perinatal period and developmental milestones should be given in infants and children presenting with history of strabismus since infancy. The clinician should be aware of common perinatal and systemic conditions associated with strabismus (Table 2.1). A family history of refractive errors and strabismus could also yield important information [1, 2]. History of previous treatment, occlusion or surgery should not be missed. Often careful inspection of old photographs of patient provide useful insight into the onset and progression of strabismus as has been discussed later in the chapter.

2.3 Assessment of Vision

Accurate assessment of vision is essential for successful management of strabismus. Assessment of fixation using torch light or brightly coloured objects in 6 weeks and older infants can provide rough idea about child's vision. Visual acuity can be assessed

S. Agrawal (✉) · A. Yadav · N. Singh
Department of Ophthalmology, King George's Medical University, Lucknow, India

© Springer Nature Singapore Pte Ltd. 2019
S. Agrawal (ed.), *Strabismus*, https://doi.org/10.1007/978-981-13-1126-0_2

in children over 2 years with some patience on E or C chart. Spending time with parents in explaining how to teach the E or C chart to the child is helpful (Fig. 2.1). Younger children would require special equipment like the preferential looking cards

Table 2.1 Common perinatal and systemic conditions associated with strabismus

• Perinatal
– Preterm delivery
– Low birth weight
– Increased maternal age
– Birth asphyxia
• Systemic
– Cerebral palsy
– Down's syndrome
– Craniofacial dysostosis

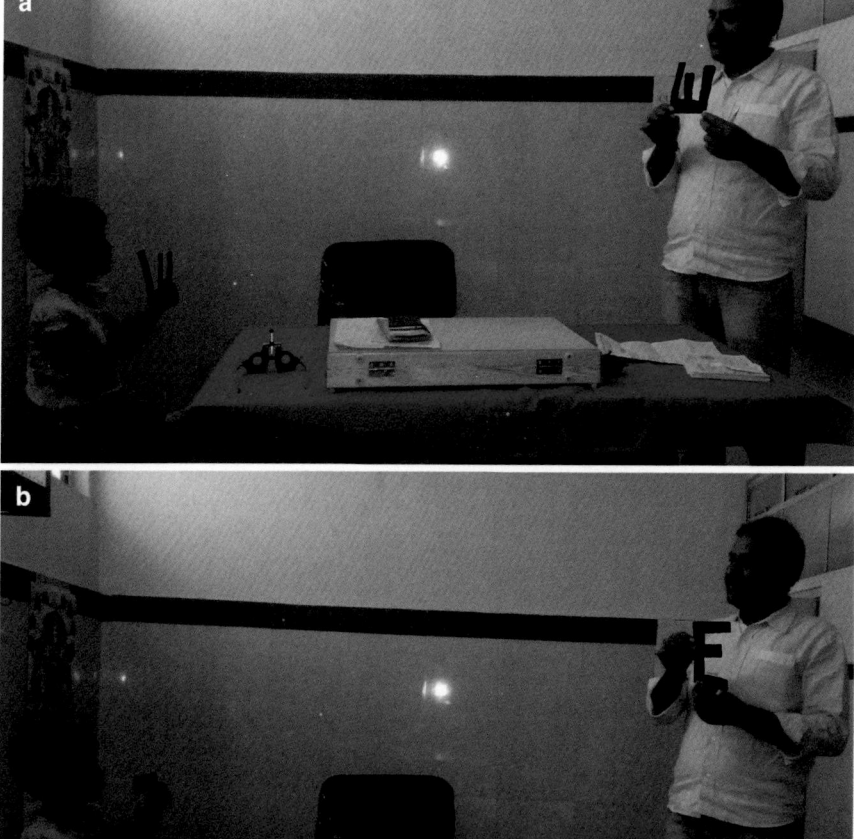

Fig. 2.1 Teaching E chart to a child

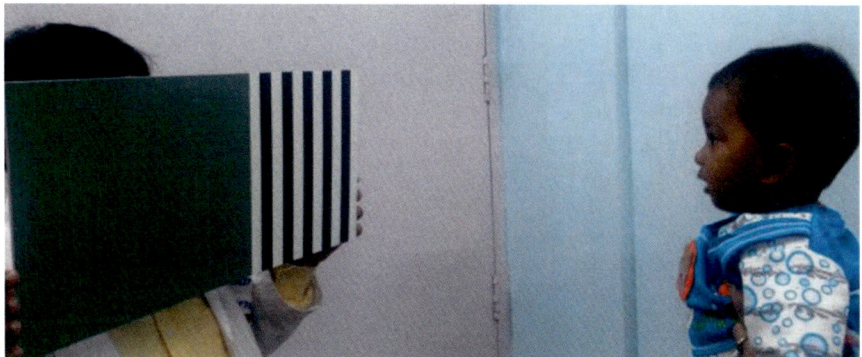

Fig. 2.2 Teller acuity cards (Stereo Optical Co, Chicago, IL) may be used to quantify visual acuity in preverbal children. They are based on the principle that the child prefers to look at the stripes rather than the blank surface. There are several cards with varying width of the stripes, and the ability to see narrower stripes denotes better acuity

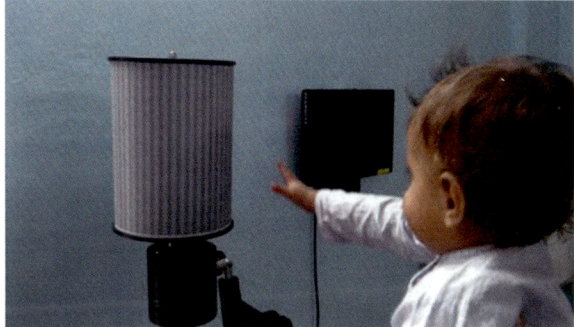

Fig. 2.3 Optokinetic drum. Nystagmus is elicited by the rotation of the drum if the child is able to visualize the gratings (lines). Gratings of the drum correspond to visual acuity, and a drum with broader gratings is used if nystagmus does not occur with finer lines

(Fig. 2.2) or the optokinetic drums (Fig. 2.3); however, a strong objection to occlusion of one eye is almost always indicative of poor vision in the other eye.

Binocular fixation preference (BFP) is a frequently used method for indirect assessment of visual acuity in children with strabismus [3]. The fixation is evaluated by making the patient fixate on an accommodative target at 40 cm with best correction in place [4]. The fixing eye is occluded forcing the other eye to take up fixation. If the eye readily takes up fixation and maintains it even after the cover is removed, the fixation pattern may be termed as central, steady, maintained (CSM). If the fixation readily shifts to the preferred eye upon the removal of occluder, the fixation is graded as central, steady, unmaintained (CSUM). If on occlusion of fixing eye, the fixation in the other eye is central but wanders off repeatedly, it is termed as central, unsteady, unmaintained (CUSUM), and if the non-preferred eye does not take up fixation at all, the fixation is termed as uncentral, unsteady, unmaintained

(UCUSUM). BFP indicates interocular difference in visual acuity, ranging from no difference in presence of CSM fixation to 0.71 ± 0.48 (LogMAR) in presence of UCUSUM [5]. If the eyes appear straight, the BFP may be checked for by covering each eye consecutively.

A better binocular vision compared to uniocular is due to binocular summation and indicates certain level of binocularity [5].

2.4   Bruckner's Test

The *Bruckner test* where the asymmetry of pupillary reflexes is observed is helpful (Fig. 2.4) in screening for deviation [6]. Taking photographs with the flash on (and red-free option in the camera set to 'off') is often helpful. Asymmetry in reflex could also be due to refractive errors or retinal pathology. Similarly, requesting the parents/patient to bring old photographs is an excellent method to confirm the duration, progression and variability of the deviation. The parents should be encouraged to take photographs of the child at different time of the day and when the child is looking at different distances.

2.5   Refraction

Cycloplegic refraction forms an essential part of strabismus examination. It assumes greater significance in children who are uncooperative for subjective visual assessment. To ensure full cycloplegia, children are often advised to come after instillations at home, and this part of examination is then completed on the second visit. Reliable assessment of motor and sensory status is only possible with the patient wearing appropriate glasses.

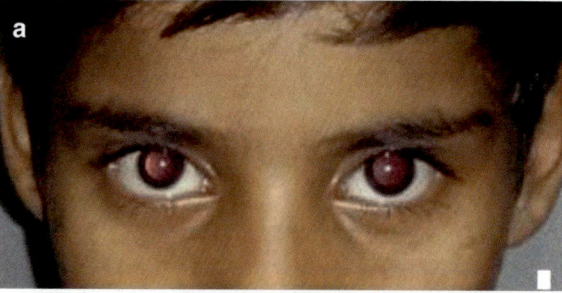
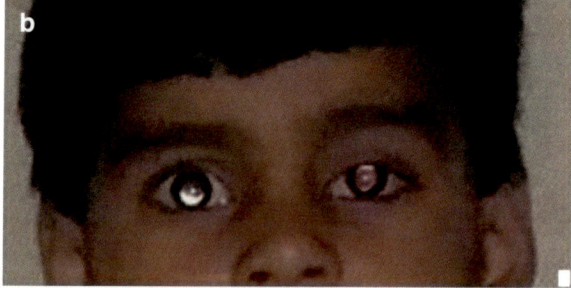

Fig. 2.4 Bruckner test showing (**a**) symmetrical reflex and (**b**) asymmetrical reflex. An asymmetrical reflex could be suggestive of anisometropia, strabismus and also of conditions like retinoblastoma, retinal detachment, media opacities, etc.

Table 2.2 Choice of cycloplegic agent

	Atropine sulphate 1% ointment	Cyclopentolate 1% eye drops	Tropicamide 0.5–0.8% + 2.5–5% phenylephrine eye drops
Indications	• First time refraction in all children <7 years or esotropic children up to 15 years • Subsequent refractions in hypermetropes up to 15 years	• First time refraction in children between 7 and 15 years or esotropic patients above 15 years • Subsequent refractions in hypermetropes over 15 years	• First time refraction above 15 years of age • Subsequent refractions in non-hypermetropes of all ages
Instillation regime	Rice grain size twice daily for 3 days	3 instillations half hour apart, 3–4 h prior	3 instillations 10 min apart, 1 h prior
Recovery	14 days	1–3 days	6–12 h

Our choice of cycloplegic agent is made according to Table 2.2 keeping in mind that the darker races require a stronger agent for longer duration compared to fairer ones.

Guidelines for prescription of glasses after refraction are discussed later. Examination of the retina should be done in the same sitting, as strabismus could be the presenting complaint of more sinister conditions like retinoblastoma [7]. At the same time one should ensure to check if the fixation is foveal. Abnormalities of fixation are not uncommon in strabismus.

2.6 Strabismus Examination

A strabismic eye is a complex product of alterations in sensory and motor mechanisms governing the physiology of the eye. Clinical examination involves detailed and systematic work up of the altered mechanisms. Basic instruments required for examination are shown in Fig. 2.5.

2.6.1 Motor Examination

The motor examination comprises of identifying the actual presence of deviation and quantifying it (both objectively and subjectively). Recognition of limitation in ocular motility, compensatory mechanisms and conditions that may mimic strabismus is also important.

2.6.1.1 Facial Symmetry and Head Posture

A thorough clinical work up begins with assessment of patient's facial features which may provide important clinical cues in understanding the underlying pathophysiology, e.g. shallow orbits and exotropia in Crouzon syndrome and hypertropia in plagiocephaly. Similarly, presence of ptosis may suggest involvement of cranial nerves, and enophthalmos may suggest a traumatic fracture of orbital floor. While studying the facial features, care must also be taken to note any anomalous head posture.

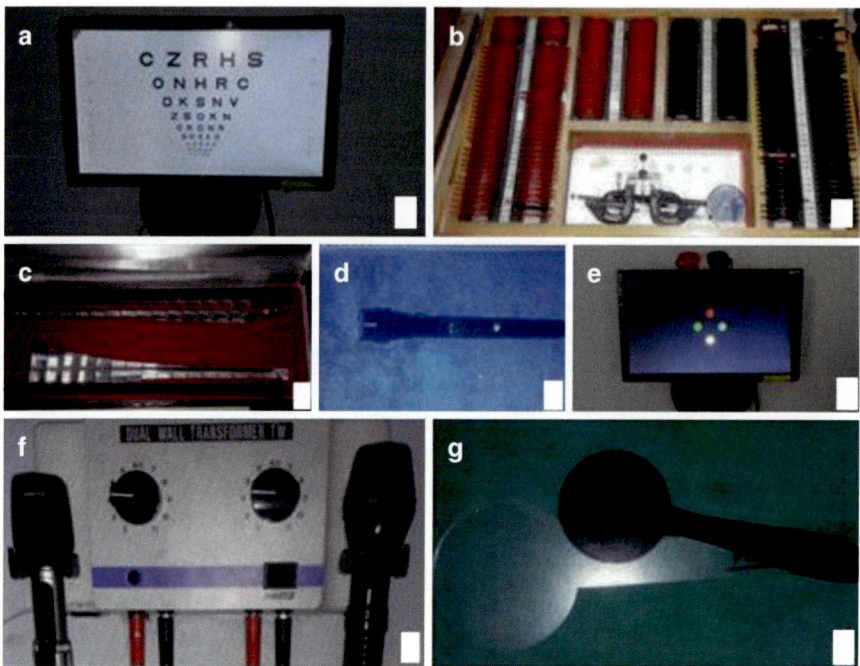

Fig. 2.5 Photograph shows basic equipment required for strabismus evaluation: (**a**) visual acuity testing chart; (**b**) trial lenses with trial frame, Lister's spot retinoscope; (**c**) horizontal and vertical prism bars; (**d**) torch; (**e**) Worth four dot test with red green glasses; (**f**) streak retinoscope and direct ophthalmoscope; (**g**) occluders. Equipment to assess sensory status like random-dot stereograms should also be available

Compensatory head postures are characteristically observed with paralytic strabismus. At the same time, it must be ensured that head posture is not merely habitual.

> **Clinical Tip**
> *When in doubt, patch one eye of the patient and observe change in head posture. Anomalous posture due to strabismus gets eliminated with closure of one eye. If it persists, a passive attempt to correct the head posture by examiner should eliminate a habitual head posture. Presence of resistance to correct posture may indicate underlying physical anomaly, e.g. torticollis.*

2.6.1.2 Assessment of Ocular Alignment

Commonly used techniques to assess ocular alignment are listed in Text Box 2.1.

Text Box 2.1: Measuring the Deviation
Objectively

- Corneal reflex test
- Prism and cover test
- Synoptophore

Subjectively

- Diplopia tests
- Haploscopic tests
- Synoptophore

Units for measurement
Degree (°): 1/360th of a circle
Prism Dioptre (*PD or* Δ): one prism dioptre prism will displace an image 1 cm at a distance of 1 m
Relation between ° *and* Δ: 1° approximately equals 2Δ (for smaller angles <40°), for larger deviations the relationship is non-linear with 45° being 100Δ and 90° being ∞
Conventionally angle is represented as '+' in esotropia and as '−' in exotropia

Hirschberg Corneal Reflex Test (HBCRT)

It is a simple yet an effective test to identify strabismus. A well-centred HBCRT is indicative of normal binocular alignment. Any decentration is usually suggestive of underlying strabismus. However, one should be careful in diagnosing strabismus only on the basis of HBCRT as decentration of reflex may be due to various other conditions like presence of a large angle kappa. A negative angle kappa may mimic esotropia, whereas a positive angle kappa may mimic exotropia [8]. Similarly, presence of prominent epicanthal folds and broad nasal bridge (Fig. 2.6) may falsely indicate presence of strabismus (pseudostrabismus) [9].

Hirschberg has demonstrated that each 1 mm decentration of corneal reflection corresponds to 7° of deviation in visual axis [10]. So, a 2 mm decentration (pupillary margin in a 4 mm pupil) would correspond to a deviation of 14°, and a 5.5 mm decentration (Limbus) would correspond to a deviation of about 40° (Fig. 2.7 and Text Box 2.2).

Krimsky Test

A simple modification of HBCRT suggested by Krimsky, in patients with blind or non-fixating one eye, is to place prisms of appropriate power in front of the fixating eye to centre the corneal reflex in the deviated eye [11].These tests have significant value in small uncooperative patients and in those undergoing purely cosmetic corrections to align a poorly seeing eye. In the latter, added benefit is inclusion of angle kappa in these measurements [8].

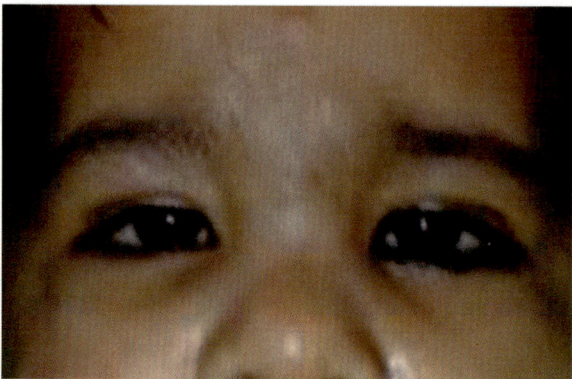

Fig. 2.6 Pseudostrabismus. Broad nasal bridge and prominent epicanthal folds give false impression of esotropia in children

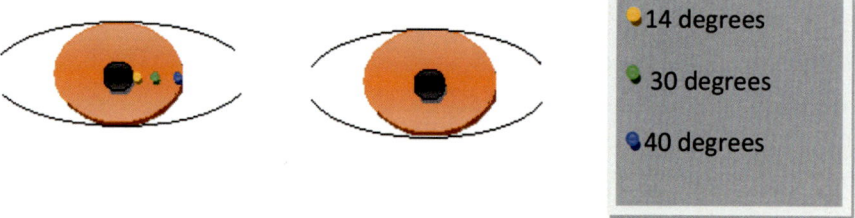

Fig. 2.7 The Hirschberg corneal reflex test

Text Box 2.2:
Documentation of deviation on Hirschberg corneal reflex test (HBCRT) is best done by drawing the corneal reflexes in relation to the pupil and the limbus, with one eye fixating at the target.

Deviation with right eye fixing on torch light (FRE)—Left Esotropia about 15°.

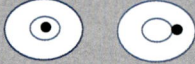

Deviation with left eye fixing on torch light (FLE)—Right Esotropia about 15°.

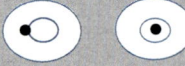

Cover and Cover-Uncover Test

As understood from the above discussion, HBCRT at best is only indicative of presence or absence of normal ocular alignment; other clinical methods are required to ascertain the presence of strabismus. Cover and cover-uncover tests are the foundations of any strabismus evaluation upon which a clinical diagnosis is reached.

Though simple and elegant, the cover test and the cover-uncover test have confused generations of residents and ophthalmologists. A systematic approach is the only key to solve 'cover and cover-uncover' puzzle, as shown in Text Box 2.3.

Clinical Tip
Cover and cover-uncover test identifies:
Strabismus from pseudostrabismus
Readiness of eyes to fixate
Phoria from tropia
Type of deviation (comitant or incomitant)
Remember: Uncover test, uncovers the phoria!

Text Box 2.3:

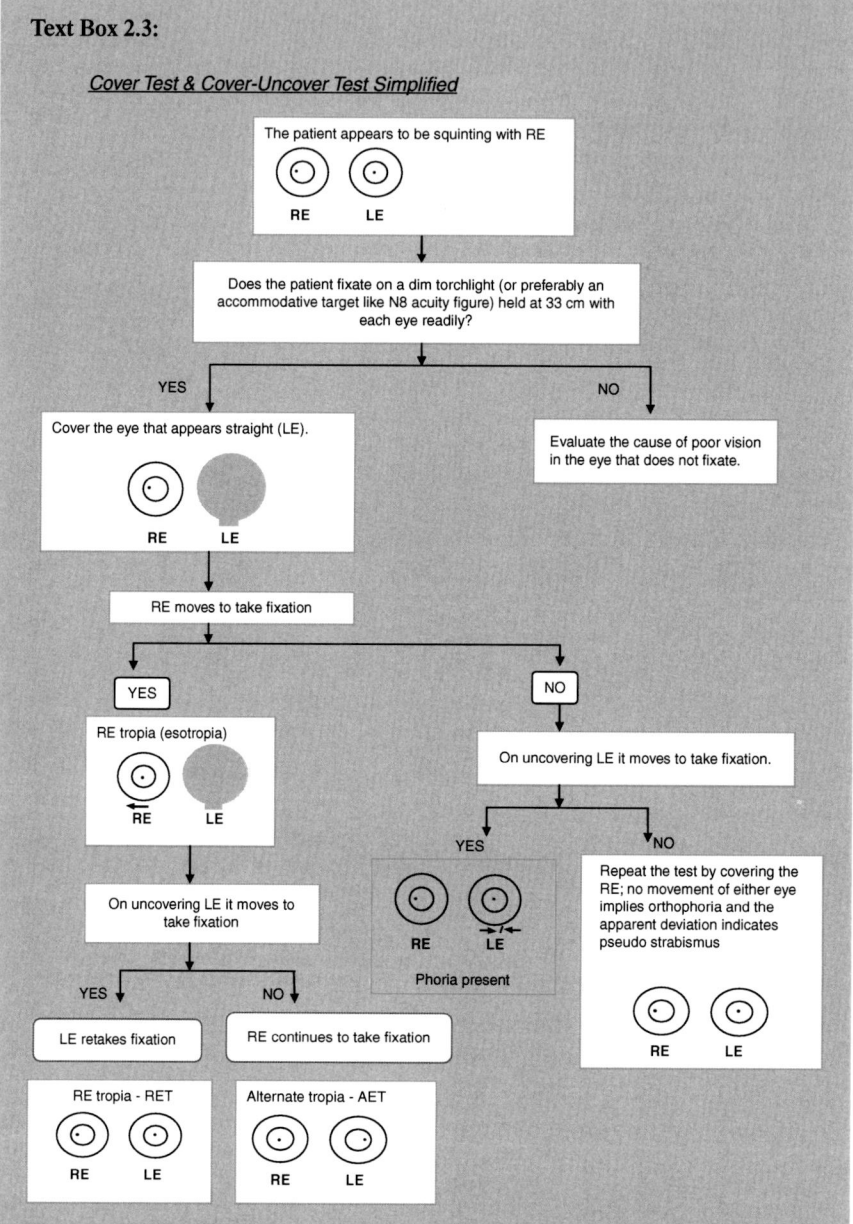

1. In the above example, outward movement of RE (esotropia) is shown. Inward movement would imply exotropia or XT. If both eyes can be made to squint, the patient has alternating tropia.
2. If movement is seen only during uncovering the eye but not during covering, it is latent squint (phoria).

3. If deviation can be demonstrated only a few times during examination, it is intermittent squint.
4. If the eye moves from out to in to take fixation, the eye has exotropia XT or exophoria X; similarly, if it moves from in to out, the eye has esotropia ET or esophoria E. Intermittent deviations are represented as X(T) or E(T), and deviation on near fixation is represented as XT′, X′, ET′ or E′.
5. Cover test should be performed both for near (33 cm) and distance (6 m) fixation.

Usually the presence or absence of deviation can be confirmed by the above test; however, if doubt persists a preliminary note should be made and the test repeated later, even on the next visit.

2.6.1.3 Measurement of Angle of Deviation

Keeping in mind that both motor and sensory mechanisms are altered in strabismus, assessment of angle of deviation may involve either measuring the angle of motor misalignment (objective assessment) or by measuring the angle of sensory malalignment of visual axis (subjective assessment). Due to presence of sensory adaptation of the visual system in presence of strabismus, the subjective assessment of angle of deviation based upon patient's subjective response to binocular stimulation may differ from objective assessment of motor malalignment.

1. *The objective assessment* of angle of deviation may be done using the following:
   (a) *Prism and Cover Test*
       Prism cover test may be performed with loose prisms or with a prism bar (prism bar and cover test (PBCT)). Alternate cover test is performed for distant and near fixation. The prism which neutralizes deviation and eliminates movement upon alternate cover test is the measurement of deviation (in prism dioptres). It is important to remember the following points while performing the prism and cover test:
   • Distance fixation should be at a target which can be easily seen. For example in a patient with visual acuity 6/6, fixation target should be at 6/9 Snellen optotype. Measurement done in this manner eliminates the effect of accommodation. Similarly, near fixation should be on an accommodative target held at 33 cm or mounted on the spectacles of examiner (Fig. 2.8).
   • It has also been recommended to measure the deviation at far distance (30 m) in patients with XT to reveal the maximum deviation [8].
   • The two eyes should be dissociated (*fusion eliminated*) to ensure that full deviation is manifest. Dissociation may be done by occlusion of one eye for 1 h to few days prior to examination. It may also be done by ensuring that patient does not regain fusion while the cover is being transferred.

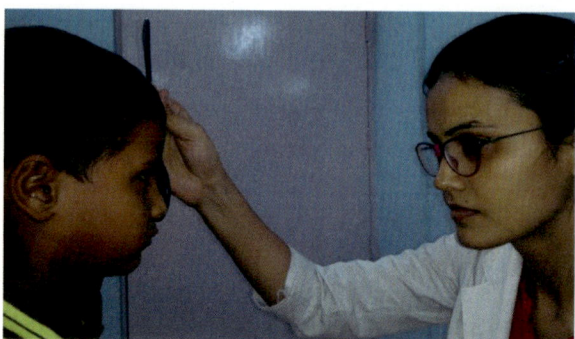

Fig. 2.8 The patient maintains near fixation on a bright-coloured sticker pasted on the spectacles of the examiner

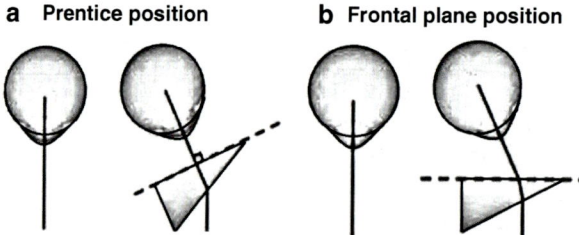

Fig. 2.9 Positioning of prisms. (**a**) Prentice position. Glass prisms are calibrated for use in this position, so the line of sight makes a right angle with one of the surfaces. (**b**) Frontal plane position. Plastic prisms are calibrated for use in this position so that the back surface lies parallel to the frontal plane of the patient

- The maximum angle of deviation should be measured by increasing the power of prisms till the direction of movement is reversed on cover test. The apex of the prisms points in the direction of deviation. For example, in ET, apex points towards the nose.
- The test should also be performed in all nine diagnostic gazes (explained in previous chapter).
- Plastic prism and bars should be held with their rear surface in frontal plane of the patient's face whereas glass prisms in Prentice position (Fig. 2.9).
- The test should be performed with either eye fixating. Initially, one eye fixates, and movement in the other eye is observed as it is alternately covered and uncovered, while a prism is placed in front of it. It is to be remembered that prisms are *not* placed over the fixating eye. The prisms are changed till the movement stops or reverses. Using the measurement of exotropia as an example, when the examiner holds a base-in prism over the right eye, the right eye is viewing in an abducted position as it looks through the prism. The left eye remains in its primary position during the measurement. Therefore, the left eye is the fixating eye during this measurement. The same is repeated with the other eye fixating.

- The measurements are same in concomitant strabismus and different in presence of incomitance where secondary deviation (deviation measured with prisms over the non-squinting eye) is larger than primary deviation (deviation measured with prisms over the primarily squinting eye). This is discussed further in Chap. 4.
- If the test is performed carefully, a difference in deviation will be noted for measurements for distance and near. It is useful to repeat the test for near after adding +3.0 D lenses to the distance correction. This would *eliminate the accommodative effort* and make the near and distance deviations almost equal.
- *The static angle of deviation should be measured after eliminating the effect of accommodation and fusion as described above.*
- *The prism and cover test has been explained in* (Fig. 2.10).

Clinical Tip

While performing Prism and cover test:

- *Eliminate head posture.*
- *Perform the test for distance (6 m) and near (33 cm) with the patient wearing appropriate correction.*
- *Never use a pen light for fixation.*
- *Use the prism over the non-fixating eye.*

(b) *Synoptophore*

Synoptophore is used to measure the angle of deviation both objectively and subjectively (Fig. 2.11). Objective angle is obtained by aligning the tubes so as to make the corneal reflection central in both eyes. Subjective angle is measured by making the patient fix alternately at a stimulus in front of each eye by alternately flashing the light in each tube. One tube is held at 0 and the other moved till there is no movement of redress of the eye that takes up fixation. The test is repeated with aligning the other tube at 0, to measure the angle fixing each eye. Horizontal, vertical and torsional deviation can be measured in different gazes. It compensates for the deviation and allows stimuli to be presented to both eyes simultaneously enabling assessment of binocular functions in the presence of heterotropia.

2. *Subjective tests* measure the deviation working on the assumption of normal retinal correspondence. In both type of tests, the eyes are dissociated by various means (like red glass, Polaroid glasses, etc.). These tests include:

    (a) *Diplopia tests* (e.g. diplopia charting, red glass test, Maddox wing) determine the subjective localisation of a single object point imaged on the fovea

Fig. 2.10 The prism and cover test. (**a**) Left esotropia. (**b**) When RE (Right Eye) is covered LE (Left Eye) moves outward to take fixation. (**c**) A base-out prism is placed in front of LE and RE is covered, there is still outward movement of LE, but amplitude of movement is decreased compared to **b**. (**d**) The cover is again transferred, and prism of greater power is held before LE. (**e**) Transfer of cover does not show movement of LE. The deviation is neutralized by prism and power of prism equals deviation

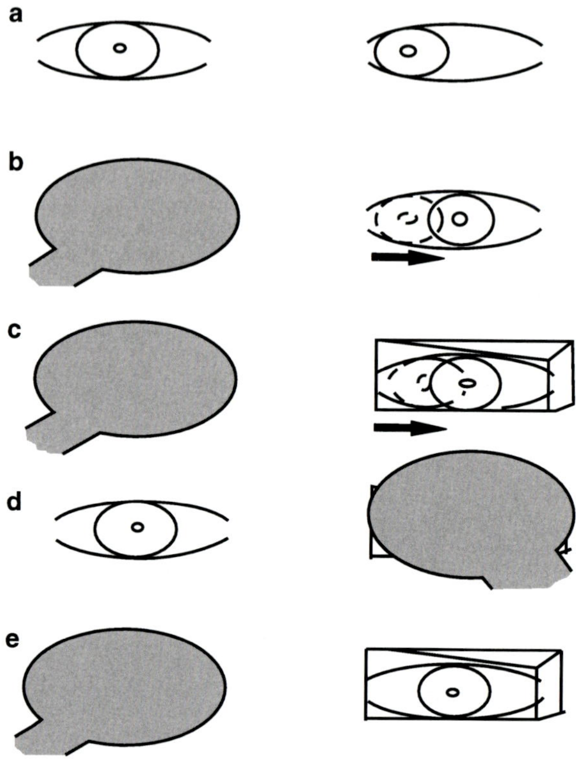

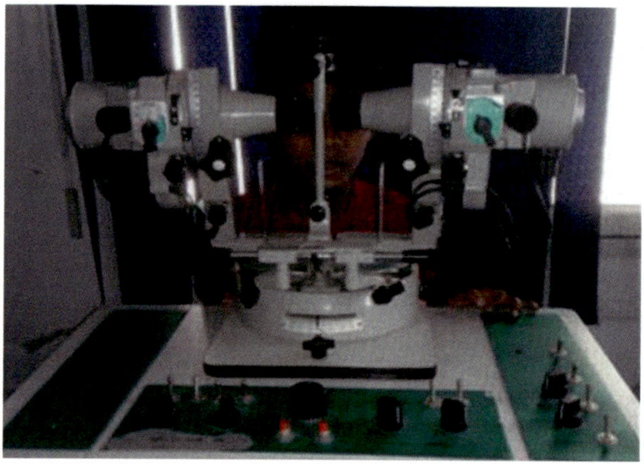

Fig. 2.11 Synoptophore

of the fixating eye and an extra foveal point in the other eye. The distance between the double images corresponds to the angle of the deviation.

(b) *Haploscopic tests* (e.g. Maddox rod, Hess charting) use two objects which are presented after dissociation of the eyes, and the patient is expected to superimpose their images (Fig. 2.12).

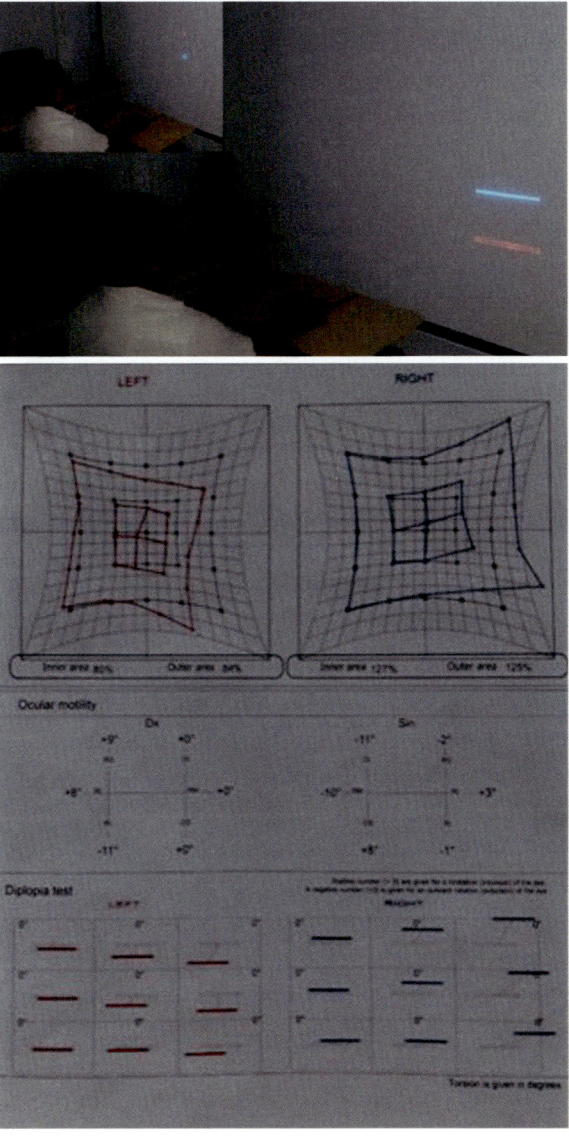

Fig. 2.12 Digital diplopia and Hess charting. The patient sits (with head posture eliminated) at 1 m from the screen wearing red filter over RE and blue filter over LE. In the above photograph, the RE sees the hollow red bar (or circle in inset image), and the LE sees the solid blue bar (or dot). The solid object is projected over different areas on the screen, and the patient moves the hollow object to surround it. The responses are representative of separation between the two images (or deviation, assuming normal retinal correspondence) seen by the patient in different gazes with the LE fixating. After a while the colour of the solid and hollow objects are interchanged to determine the deviation with RE fixating. The machine output in cranial nerve III paresis is shown

2.6.1.4 Motility

Uniocular and binocular motility assessment is an essential component of strabismus work up. Basic features of uniocular movements (ductions), synchronous simultaneous movements of both eyes in same direction (versions) and fusional movements (vergences) have been discussed in the previous chapter.

For ductions, one eye is covered, and the patient is asked to follow a fixation target with the other eye to the farthest possible position in different directions and a limitation of motility noted. For versions, similarly the patient is asked to follow the fixation target with both eyes, starting from midline. The distance of the target is so maintained that both eyes are able to see it at all times. Movement of both the eyes are thus compared.

Functional motility is demonstrated by versions and is hence more important [12]. Ductions demonstrate the maximum movement possible with the strongest innervational impulse. A limited duction is usually due to a significant muscle palsy or mechanical restriction. Versions are tested in the six cardinal gazes (as elaborated in the previous chapter) in each of which a pair of muscles (yoke muscles) are maximally contracting. If it is possible to identify the gaze with maximal motility limitation and diplopia, the deviation can be attributed to the pair of muscles contracting in it [13, 14].

Photographs demonstrating motility limitation should be kept in records (Fig. 2.13). Grading of ocular motility is discussed in detail in Chap. 4.

> **Clinical Tip**
> *Once versions are tested, the uniocular motility (ductions) should always be tested.*

Amongst vergences, fusional convergence and divergence are of clinical relevance to the general ophthalmologist. While fusional convergence helps to control an exophoria, fusional divergence controls an esophoria. The normal range for convergence is 15Δ for distance and about 35Δ for near; for divergence is 6Δ for distance and about 15Δ for near [15].Amplitudes are measured by prisms or synoptophore. These may be reduced by fatigue or illness thereby converting a phoria into tropia and may be improved by orthoptic exercises.

The near point of convergence (NPC) is normally about 8–10 cm [8]. It may be measured by placing a fixation target at about 30–40 cm in the midplane of the patient's head. The patient maintains fixation on the object as it is moved towards him. The distance at which either eye loses fixation and moves out is the objective NPC, and the point at which the patient complains of diplopia or blurring is the subjective NPC. The objective NPC is more proximal, i.e. diplopia occurs prior to the deviation of the eye. An NPC further than 10 cm is remote and may be up to 30 cm in patients with convergence insufficiency [8]. Near point of accommodation (NPA) is the nearest point on which the eyes maintain clear focus, and it recedes with age.

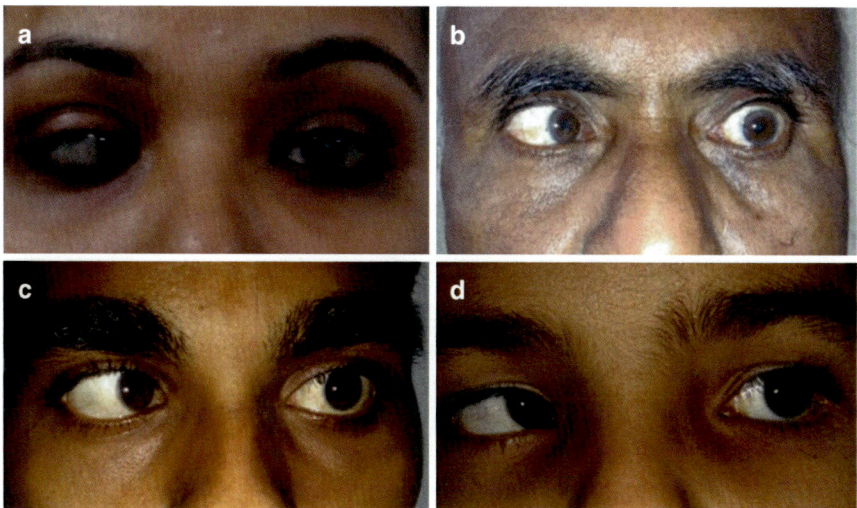

Fig. 2.13 Grading reduced ocular motility (versions). In these photographs limited movement of left eye in levoversion is being demonstrated. (**a**) Severe, not crossing the midline; (**b**) moderate, just crossing the midline; (**c**) mild; (**d**) almost full

2.6.2 Examination of the Sensory State

Assessment of sensory alterations in strabismus is as important as motor examination because it gives an insight into the eventual prognosis of the patient. Sensory state evaluation is even more imperative amongst children as corrective measures to improve sensory alterations during the period of visual immaturity may improve the motor alterations. It is also important during follow-up of patients as the ultimate goal of strabismus management is to provide near normal sensory status to the patient, i.e. binocular single vision with good stereopsis. Sensory examination of a patient with strabismus comprises of determining the binocular state with various possibilities like (1) diplopia, (2) suppression, (3) abnormal retinal correspondence or (4) stereopsis. It also involves examination for amblyopia, a condition which persists even after occlusion of the fixating eye.

During follow-up visits, the sensory assessment may take precedence over the other tests done monocularly (like vision assessment) as they may disrupt the fusional control in some patients.

2.6.2.1 Diplopia Charting

Before proceeding with examination in a patient with diplopia, it should be confirmed whether the patient is actually meaning double vision or he is confusing some other symptom with it. It should also be determined whether the diplopia is uniocular or binocular.

Diplopia in strabismus is binocular and usually a feature of incomitant deviation. It may be *uncrossed* as in ET with the image corresponding to each eye forming on the same side, i.e. right eye image on the right side of the patient or *crossed* as in XT. It may also be vertical or torsional. Diplopia charting is done using red and green filters with the patient looking at a fixation light and reporting the subjective positions of the two light images seen. Conventionally red filter is used over the right eye (Fig. 2.14). Care must be taken to eliminate the anomalous head posture, accurately chart the location of the images and separation between them in different gazes. Maximum separation of images occurs in the gaze of action of the paralyzed muscle with the farther image belonging to the eye with paralysis.

> **Clinical Tip**
> *To detect the paralyzed muscle on diplopia chart, note must be made of the following:*
>
> - *Type of diplopia*
> - *Gaze of maximum diplopia*
> - *Colour of the farther image*

2.6.2.2 Suppression

Suppression has been defined and briefly explained in the previous chapter. A patient with good vision in both eyes and not having diplopia in the presence of long-standing heterotropia is invariably suppressing the image from one eye. In central suppression the image from foveal area of the deviating eye is suppressed, and the corresponding depression in binocular single field is termed as the suppression scotoma. The area of this scotoma can be determined by using prisms to shift the image out of this area to induce diplopia.

Worth four dot test (WFDT) is also used for diagnosing suppression (Fig. 2.15). The test should be performed both for near and distance. Deviation should be assessed (by cover test) after the patient wears red green glasses, as intermittent deviations with unstable binocularity may become manifest as the eyes dissociate [16, 17]. This may require to make the patient wear prisms to compensate for the deviation before proceeding with interpretation of the WFDT.

Fig. 2.14 *Diplopia charting* with red filter (represented by solid line) over the right eye in a patient with left lateral rectus palsy   Dextroversion 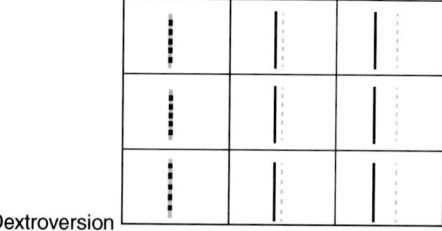 Levoversion

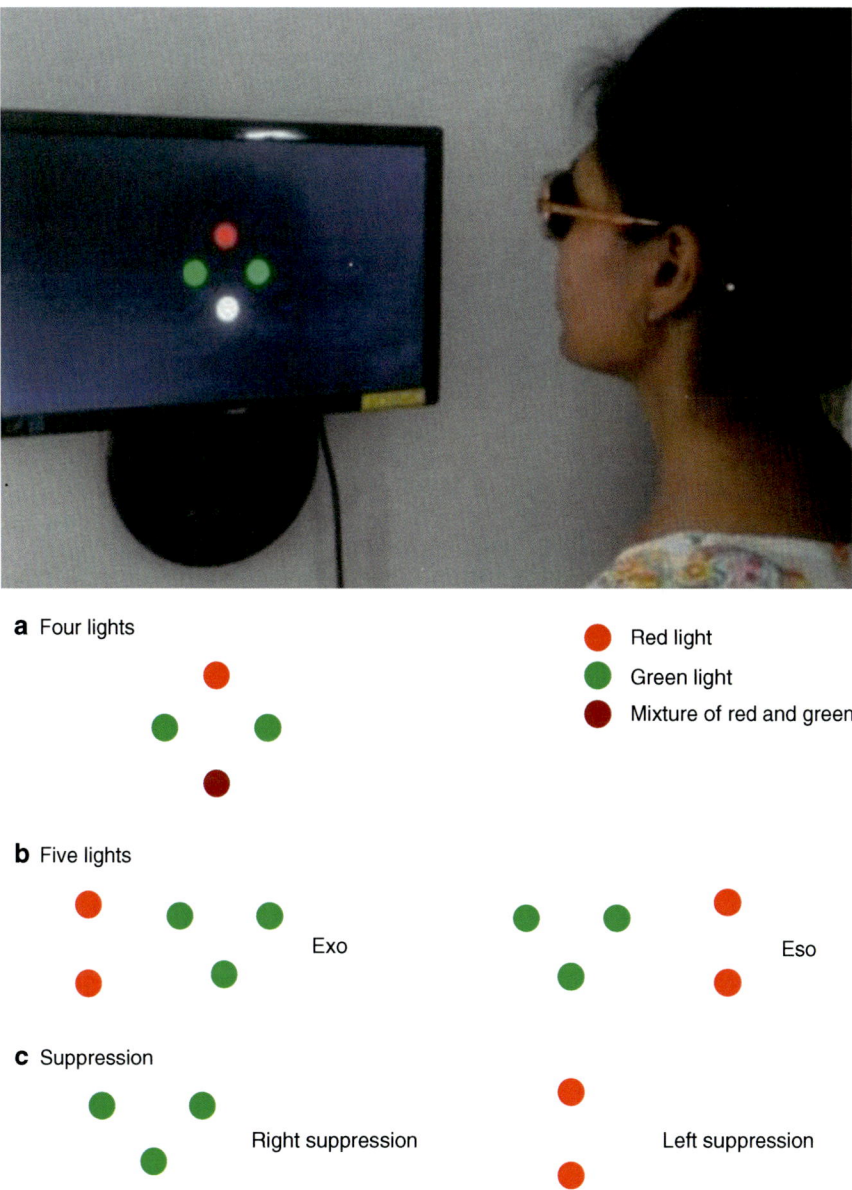

Fig. 2.15 *Worth four dot test* should be performed at 6 m and 33 cm distance. Interpretation according to what the patient sees. (**a**) Four lights (one red, two green and one light that is a mixture of red and green)—fusion with orthotropia. (**b**) Five lights—diplopia with deviation. The lights are displaced according to the type of deviation present. Red lights are seen on the left (crossed diplopia) in XT and on the right (uncrossed diplopia) in ET. (**c**) Three or two lights—suppression. Three green lights indicate right eye suppression, and two red lights indicate left eye suppression. Note: Interpretation (**a**) may also occur in presence of a small-angle deviation with abnormal retinal correspondence (ARC)

2.6.2.3 Abnormal Retinal Correspondence (ARC)

ARC has also been introduced in the previous chapter. It should be suspected in long-standing, early-onset, small-angle, constant esotropia when the objective and the subjective angle measurements do not coincide. It should also be suspected when binocularity is observed in presence of obvious deviation.

Several methods have been described to test for ARC of which striated glasses of Bagolini and foveo-foveal test of Cuppers are easy to perform and give necessary information [18, 19]. In a simplified version of the latter test, the examiner projects the asterisk of the visuscope attachment of the direct ophthalmoscope onto the fovea of the deviated eye, while the other eye fixates on a fixation light. In presence of normal retinal correspondence, the asterisk and the fixation light would appear superimposed to the patient and which would not be the case in the presence of ARC. If the fixation light is mounted on a device like the Maddox cross, the amount of ARC (or the angle of anomaly) can be determined.

ARC is not treated in adults as treatment may make an otherwise asymptomatic patient develop intractable diplopia [20].

2.6.2.4 Amblyopia

Amblyopia is unilateral or, less frequently, bilateral reduction in best corrected visual acuity, in the absence of any identifiable pathology of the eye or visual pathway. It is attributed to failure of normal neural development in the immature visual system due to form vision deprivation and/or abnormal binocular interaction in early in life [21].Its causes are strabismus, refractive errors and visual deprivation due to conditions like ptosis, corneal opacities, cataract, etc. In a child with diminished vision, the diagnosis of amblyopia should be one of exclusion.

Common signs in amblyopia are (1) in presence of strabismus, the non-amblyopic eye has a strong *preference to take up fixation*; (2) visual *acuity* of the amblyopic eye is reduced; (3) *colour, contrast* and *accommodation* are reduced; (4) *crowding phenomenon* occurs, where acuity when measured with single letters is better compared to conventional charts; (5) visual acuity improves under *mesopic* conditions; (6) eccentric fixation may occur; and (7) abnormalities of pupillary reaction and pursuits may occur.

Confirmation and quantification of amblyopia may require multiple assessments. Principles of treatment involve elimination of the cause, correction of refractive error and forcing the use of amblyopic eye. Details are discussed later.

2.6.2.5 Stereopsis

Restoring normal stereopsis is the ultimate goal of strabismus treatment. In presence of strabismus, presence of stereoscopic vision in any part of binocular field carries good prognosis to treatment [22]. Considering this, testing for stereopsis should always be done after the deviation has been corrected surgically or compensated for by prisms or synoptophore.

Numerous tests have been described for testing stereopsis but all have the same principle, i.e. dissociation of the two eyes (each eye is presented a separate field of view), and each of the two fields contain elements that stimulate corresponding retinal points. This enables fusion of the disparate images enabling stereoscopic vision. We discuss the commonly used tests.

Two-pencil test (Fig. 2.16) is a simple method to test gross stereopsis [23, 24]. We have found this test particularly useful to explain to the parents the utility of binocular vision and to motivate them for early surgery.

Synoptophore as already discussed compensates for the deviation and also dissociates both the eyes by mechanically separated fields of view. The targets are interchangeable and set optically at infinity by use of suitable lenses. Binocular vision is graded on synoptophore (Fig. 2.17) as:

1. *First grade—simultaneous macular perception (SMP)*, tested by one slide seen foveally (like a joker) and the other seen parafoveally (like a hut). A patient having SMP would perceive the joker inside the hut.

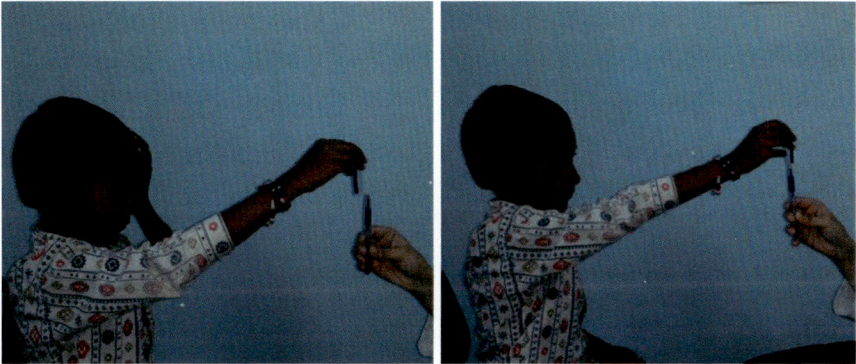

Fig. 2.16 A modification of the two-pencil test requires the patient to cap a pen (held by the examiner) with an out stretched hand. This simple manoeuver becomes difficult in the absence of stereopsis or with one eye closed

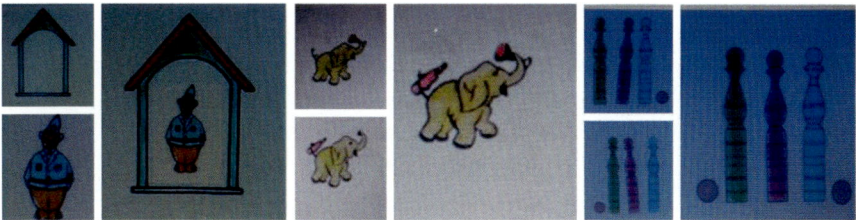

Fig. 2.17 Binocular vision on synoptophore. (L to R) SMP, fusion and stereopsis tested on the synoptophore. The two images on left in each show the slides projected individually to each eye, and the larger image shows its normal binocular visualization. In presence of stereopsis, the central wicket is seen placed posterior to the lateral ones, and two balls on either side are used to confirm if the patient is actually seeing the image with both the eyes

Fig. 2.18 Randot stereoacuity test. The patient wears a Polaroid glass and recognizes the objects that appear to project above the surface

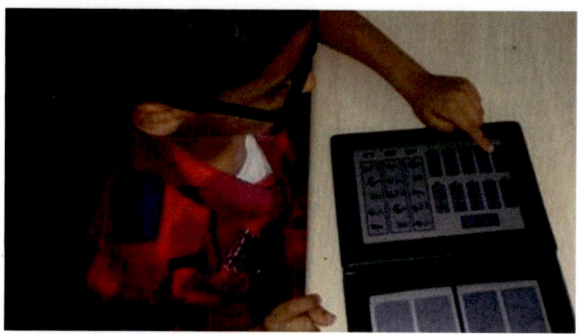

2. *Second grade—fusion*, tested by similar but incomplete pictures which the patient with intact sensory fusion would perceive as single and complete. Ability to maintain fusion (motor fusion) in convergence and divergence is tested by moving the arms of the synoptophore.
3. *Third grade—stereopsis*, tested by pictures of the same object taken from slightly different angles which an individual with stereopsis would perceive in depth.

In other tests, polarized glasses are used to dissociate the eyes, with superimposed stereoscopic images so printed on the test card that only one image is seen exclusively with each eye. *Titmus stereo* test is for gross stereopsis, *Random Dot E* test is used for screening and the *Randot* test (Fig. 2.18) is the current test of choice in the clinic as it almost eliminates the monocular clues and quantifies stereopsis upto 20 s of arc [25, 26]. Distance stereopsis assessment is also important especially in intermittent exotropia patients in whom fusion at distance is often compromised. A reducing distance stereopsis may be considered as poor control and warrant surgical correction. Distance stereoacuity may be tested using Frisby Davis Distance (FD2) and Distance Randot test [27, 28].

2.7 Few Other Important Concepts

Binocular potential score is a scoring system to predict the postoperative outcome in horizontal concomitant strabismus. It takes into account the preoperative factors like age of onset, duration, intermittency, variability, vision and responses on synoptophore and Worth four dot test [28].

Ocular dominance is the tendency to prefer visual input from one eye to the other [29]. A simple test to determine it is to view an object with both eyes open through a pinhole held with extended arms. The pinhole is then brought close to face keeping the object in view, and it eventually covers the dominant eye. As will be discussed later, determining the dominant eye is important in surgical planning.

Sample of our strabismus case sheet is attached as Annexure 1.

2.8 Summary

- Strabismus could be the presenting complaint of a serious disease like retinoblastoma.
- Clinical evaluation of strabismus involves a systematic and step-by-step approach beginning from eliciting relevant clinical history to the assessment of motor and sensory status.
- Any refractive error should be corrected before proceeding with strabismus evaluation.
- Cover and cover-uncover test are basic foundations of strabismus evaluation.
- Objective assessment of angle of deviation is done by prism and cover test. Deviation should be assessed in all gazes with either eye fixating. Assessment should be done both for near and distance fixation.
- Binocular movement (versions) assessment is essential to evaluate under- and overaction of extraocular muscles. Uniocular movement (ductions) should always be checked before considering paralytic or restrictive strabismus.
- The ocular deviation should be neutralized using prisms before assessing binocular sensory state.
- Tests for diplopia, suppression, stereopsis and abnormal retinal correspondence constitute binocular sensory state assessment.
- Binocular sensory state assessment is indispensable to strabismus examination and should also be done during follow-up visits.

2.9 Multiple Choice Questions

1. Krimsky test is useful in the following setting:
   (a) Measuring deviation in young uncooperative children
   (b) Sensory exotropia
   (c) Sensory esotropia
   (d) All of the above

Answer: (d) Krimsky test has significant value in small uncooperative patients and in those undergoing purely cosmetic corrections to align a poorly seeing eye.

2. Cycloplegic of choice for first time refraction in a 2-year-old Indian child with suspected esotropia is:
   (a) Eye drop cyclopentolate, three installations half hour apart, 3–4 h prior
   (b) Eye drop tropicamide + phenylephrine three installations 10 min apart, 1 h prior
   (c) Atropine eye drop two installations 12 h apart from 1 day prior
   (d) Atropine eye ointment 12 hourly installations from 3 day prior

Answer: (d) Atropine is the cycloplegic agent of choice in all children below 7 years and in children with esotropia up to 15 years. It has to be used for 3 days. Atropine eye ointment is preferred as it has lesser systemic absorption.

3. Which amongst the following tests is *not* used to assess the binocular functions?
   (a) Random dot
   (b) Worth four dot
   (c) Hirschberg
   (d) Synoptophore

Answer: (c) Hirschberg corneal reflex test is used to assess the ocular deviation.

4. Which is the best grade of binocular vision?
   (a) Stereopsis
   (b) Simultaneous macular perception
   (c) Suppression
   (d) Fusion

Answer: (a) Suppression implies absence of binocular vision. Other two are inferior grades compared to stereopsis.

5. Which of the following is a prerequisite for performing cover test and cover-uncover test?
   (a) Vision in both eyes should be nearly equal
   (b) Both eyes should be able to fixate at the target
   (c) Prism bar or loose prisms should be available
   (d) The patient should be literate

Answer: (b) Equal vision is not required, but it should be enough in each to enable fixation on the target being used. Prisms are required for prism and cover test to neutralize the deviation.

References

1. Birch EE, Fawcett SL, Morale SE, Weakley DR, Wheaton DH. Risk factors for accommodative esotropia among hypermetropic children. Invest Ophthalmol Vis Sci. 2005;46:526–9.
2. Mohney BG. Common forms of childhood esotropia. Ophthalmology. 2001;108:805–9.
3. Kutschke P. Preverbal assessment of amblyopia. Am Orthop J. 2005;55:53–61.
4. Kothari M, Bhaskare A, Mete D, Toshniwal S, Doshi P, Kaul S. Evaluation of central, steady, maintained fixation grading for predicting inter-eye visual acuity difference to diagnose and treat amblyopia in strabismic patients. Indian J Ophthalmol. 2009;57:281–4.
5. Azen SP, Varma R, Preston-Martin S, Ying-Lai M, Globe D, Hahn S. Binocular visual acuity summation and inhibition in an ocular epidemiological study: the Los Angeles Latino eye study. Invest Ophthalmol Vis Sci. 2002;43:1742–8.

6. American Academy of Pediatrics, American Association of Pediatric Ophthalmology and Strabismus, and the American Academy of Ophthalmology. Eye examination in infants, children and young adults by pediatricians. Pediatrics. 2003;111:902–7.
7. Balmer A, Munier F. Differential diagnosis of leukocoria and strabismus, first presenting signs of retinoblastoma. Clin Ophthalmol. 2007;1:431–9.
8. Von Noorden GK, Campos EC. Chapter 12: Examination of the patient II. In: Binocular vision and ocular motility. 6th ed. St. Louis: Mosby; 2002. p. 168–210.
9. Kanski JJ, Strabismus BB. Clinical ophthalmology: a systematic approach. 8th ed. Philadelphia: Elsevier Health Sciences; 2011. p. 755–6.
10. Hirschberg J. Uber die Messundg des SChielgrades und die Dosierung der Schielopeartion. Zentralbl Prakt Augenkeilkd. 1885;9:325.
11. Krimskey E. The binocular examination of the young child. Am J Ophthalmol. 1943;26:624.
12. Bielschowsky A. Lectures on motor anomalies. Hannover, NH: Dartmouth College Publications; 1943/1956.
13. Hering E. The teaching of the binocular. Leipzig: Wilhelm Engelmann; 1868.
14. Sherrington CS. Experimental note on two movements of the eye. J Physiol Lond. 1894;17:27.
15. Berens C, Losey CC, Hardy LH. Routine examination of the ocular muscles and non-operative treatment. Am J Ophthalmol. 1927;10:910.
16. Von Noorden GK, Campos EC. Chapter 13: Examination of the patient III. In: Binocular vision and ocular motility. 6th ed. St. Louis: Mosby; 2002. p. 211–45.
17. von Noorden GK. Infantile esotropia: A continuing riddle (Scobee Lecture). Am Orthopt J. 1984;34:52.
18. Bagolini B. Technica per Iésame della vision binoculare sense introduzione di elementi dissocianti: "test del vetro striato". Boll Ocul. 1958;37:195.
19. Cuppers C. Moderne Schielbehandlung. Klin Monatsbl Augenheilkd. 1956;129:579.
20. Quere MA, Lavenant G, Pechereau A, et al. Les diplopies incoercibles post-therapeutiques. J Fr Orthopt. 1993;25:191.
21. Cantor LB, Rapuano CJ, Cioffi GA. Chapter 4. Amblyopia. In: Section 6. Basic and clinical science course 2015–16. San Francisco: American Academy of Ophthalmology. p. 33–40.
22. Von Noorden GK, Campos EC. Chapter 15: Examination of the patient V. In: Binocular vision and ocular motility. 6th ed. St. Louis: Mosby; 2002. p. 298–307.
23. Lang J. Der Treffversuch zur Prufung des stereoskopischen Sehens. Klin Monatsbl Augenheilkd. 1974;165:895.
24. LaRoche R, von Norrden GK. Theoretical and practical evaluation of a simple stereotest. Invest Ophthalmol Vis Sci. 1982;22(Suppl):266.
25. Fawcett SL, Birch EE. Interobserver test-retest reliability of the Randot preschool stereoacuity test. J Am Assoc Pediatr Ophthalmol Strabismus. 2000;4:354–8.
26. Fricke TR, Siderov J. Stereopsis, stereotests, and their relation to vision screening and clinical practice. Clin Exp Optom. 1997;80(5):165–72.
27. Holmes JM, Birch EE, Mohney BG. Newer test of distance stereoacuity and their role in evaluating intermittent exotropia. Ophthalmology. 2007;114(6):1215–20.
28. Singh V, Pandey M, Agrawal S. Binocular potential score: a novel concept. J Pediatr Ophthalmol Strabismus. 2008;45(2):104–8.
29. Khan AZ, Crawford JD. Ocular dominance reverses as a function of horizontal gaze angle. Vis Res. 2001;41(14):1743–8.

Annexure 1: Sample Strabismus Case Sheet

Patient's name
Age   **Sex**   **Occupation**
Address & Phone
Orthoptic Clinic registration number
Date of 1st Visit
Chief complaints

Brief history

Other relevant history
Family/Trauma/Perinatal/Past Treatment/Systemic
Findings on old photographs

Vision	With glasses		Without glasses		Glasses No.	Near vision with + 3.0 for amblyopes
	Distance	Near	Distance	Near		
RE						
LE						

Using glasses since
Present glasses since
Retinoscopy   (Atropine/Cyclopentolate/Tropicamide/without cycloplegia)

Deviation under cycloplegia
Fundus
Fixation
Any other ocular finding

Motor Assessment
1. **Anomalous head posture (AHP):** (a) Face   (b) Chin   (c) Head
2. **Primary Ocular Direction:**   With glasses   without glasses

3. **Ocular Deviation**
   (by Hirschberg Corneal Reflex)   FLE ⊙⊙   FRE ⊙⊙

4. **Cover test**
   (a)   Nature of Deviation
       • Orthotropia
       • Phoria X or E
       • Tropia X(T), X(T)', XT, XT'
           – E(T), E(T)', ET, ET'
           – Preferential Fixation RE/LE/Either Eye

   (b)   Amount of Deviation (confirmed with PCT)
   - FRE
   - FLE
   - Change without glasses
   - Change from up to downgaze
   - Near/distance disparity
   - AC/A ratio

5. **Ocular movements**
   (a) Versions   (b) Limitation in ductions

DV
LV

6. **Proximal convergence** (a) Objective   (b) Subjective

Sensory Assessment
   1. **Synoptophore**
       (a) Simultaneous Macular Perception Yes/No
       (b) Fusion obtained at: (+):   maintained till: recovery at:
                                   (−):
       (c) Stereopsis   Yes/No
       (d)

Angle	Subjective	Objective (by corneal reflex)*
FLE		
FRE		

                              *Actually a part of motor assessment

   2. **Worth Four Dot Test**
   3. **Randot Stereoacuity** (a) Near   (b) Distance
   4. **Diplopia Chart**
       (a)

DV
LV

       (b) Quadrant of maximum diplopia

   5. **Hess Chart**

Diagnosis/Differentials

Special scores/tests for management planning & prognosis
1. Binocular Potential Score
2. Newcastle Control Score or Mayo Clinic Score for X(T)
3. Prism Adaptation Test (a) Deviation
                             (b) Binocularity
4. Axial Length   RE   LE

Management Plan

Follow-up

(Abbreviations: *FLE* fixating with left eye, *FRE* fixating with right eye, *X* exophoria, *E* esophoria, *X(T)* intermittent exotropia, *X(T)'* intermittent exotropia for near, *XT* exotropia, *XT'* exotropia for near, *E(T)* intermittent esotropia, *E(T)'* intermittent esotropia for near, *ET* esotropia, *ET'* esotropia for near, *PCT* prism and cover test, *AC/A* Accommodative convergence/Accommodation, *DV* dextroversion, *LV* levoversion)

Comitant Horizontal Strabismus

3

Siddharth Agrawal, Rajat M. Srivastava, and Ankur Yadav

3.1   Introduction

Horizontal comitant strabismus forms the single largest group of strabismus we encounter routinely. In spite of their clinical abundance, varied presentation makes this subtype challenging even for an experienced observer.

Broadly speaking, a horizontal comitant deviation could be either esotropia (ET) or exotropia (XT) depending on whether either eye deviates inwards (nasally) or outwards (temporally). The literal meaning of 'committance' is to be pledged or to accompany in a subordinate way. Both the eyes (are pledged to each other and) have equal deviation in all directions of gaze for a given fixation distance. The seat of anomaly is usually the brain unlike incomitant deviations which arise out of defect in the neuro muscular complex.

Dynamic mechanisms (e.g. accommodation, fusional vergence) may be superimposed or may mask the deviation. Residents often confuse esotropia to be the opposite of exotropia; however, they should be considered as totally different entities.

A simplified classification of ET and XT is mentioned in Table 3.1.

3.2   Esotropia and Its Management

A number of anomalies may lead to esotropia (Fig. 3.1), and it is essential to elaborate the underlying pathophysiology in order to administer the appropriate treatment.

Before going into the types of ET, it would be worthwhile to talk about esophoria E and intermittent esotropia E(T), both of which are usually compensated by

S. Agrawal (✉) · R. M. Srivastava · A. Yadav
Department of Ophthalmology, King George's Medical University, Lucknow, India

© Springer Nature Singapore Pte Ltd. 2019
S. Agrawal (ed.), *Strabismus*, https://doi.org/10.1007/978-981-13-1126-0_3

Table 3.1 Simplified classification of comitant horizontal deviations

Esodeviations
1. Accommodative
Refractive
Non-refractive
Hyperaccommodative (high AC/A)
Hypoaccommodative (reduced NPA)
Partially accommodative
2. Nonaccommodative
Essential infantile
Late onset
Basic type
Acute onset
Convergence excess
3. Sensory
4. Less frequent types
Cyclic[a]
Microtropia
NBS[a]
ET with neurological abnormalities
Exodeviations
1. X
2. X(T)
3. XT
Divergence excess
Basic
Convergence insufficiency
Simulated divergence excess
4. Sensory

ET esotropia, *XT* exotropia, *X* exophoria, *X(T)* intermittent exotropia, *AC/A* accommodative convergence/accommodation, *NPA* near point of accommodation, *NBS* nystagmus blockage syndrome
[a]Discussed in other chapters

Fig. 3.1 Esotropia left eye

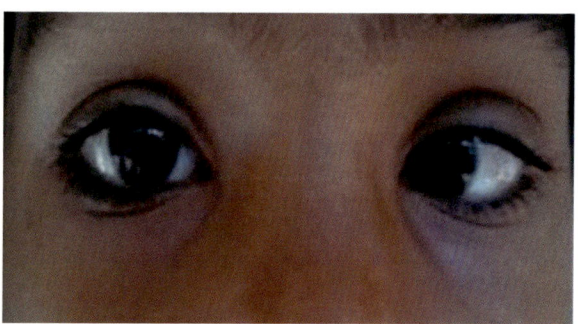

fusional reserves. Refractive correction should be done. If the asthenopia persists, the patient should be referred to a specialist to consider a trial of prisms or, in rare cases, surgery. The following discussion outlines basic characteristics and management of various subtypes of esotropia.

3.2.1 Accommodative ET

Accommodative ET is caused by increased accommodative effort or an abnormally high accommodative convergence/accommodation (AC/A) ratio. Its onset is usually between 2 and 3 years of age, and the deviation for near fixation is larger than that for distance [1]. Simplified approach to diagnosis and management of accommodative ET is represented in Table 3.2.

1. *Refractive accommodative ET* is due to uncorrected hypermetropia. ET occurs because of convergence associated with persistent accommodative effort to overcome uncorrected hypermetropia. AC/A ratio is normal, and it is fully corrected in all gazes and at all fixation distances by refractive correction.

Table 3.2 Diagnosis and management of accommodative esotropia

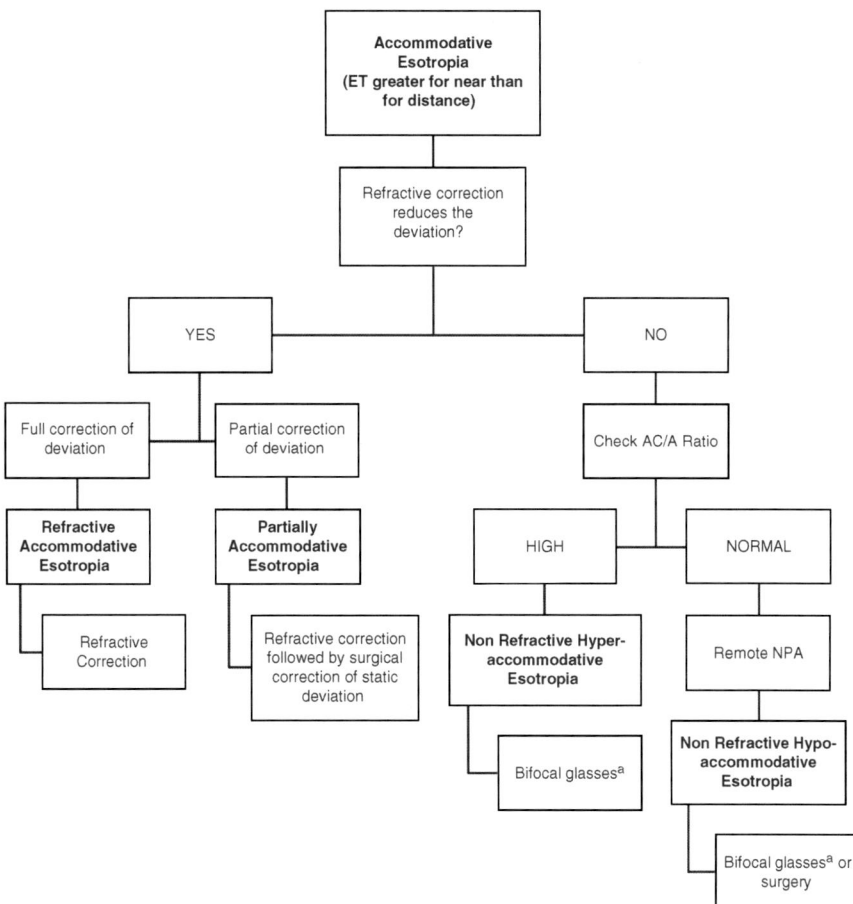

AC/A accommodative convergence/accommodation, *ET* esotropia, *NPA* near point of accommodation

[a]Bifocal glasses should eliminate the near deviation and have no utility if the deviation merely reduces

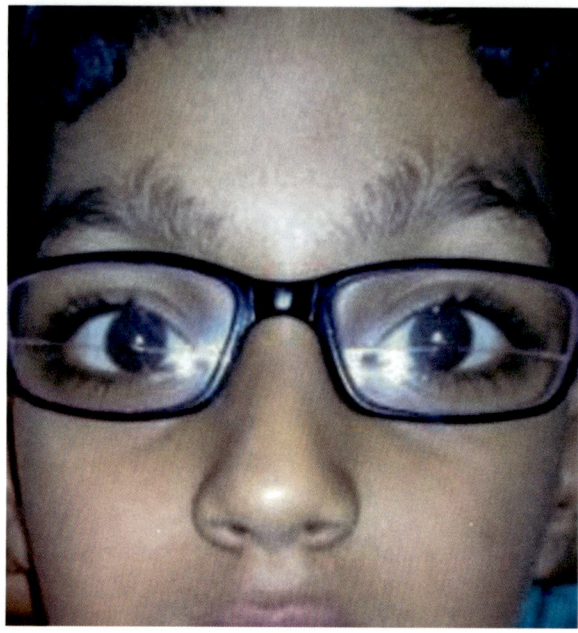

Fig. 3.2 Pupil bisecting executive bifocals

2. *Non-refractive hyperaccommodative ET* is caused by an abnormally high accommodative convergence/accommodation (AC/A) ratio with a normal near point of accommodation. The deviation is greater for near fixation and is unrelated to the refractive error. It is treated by prescribing straight top (executive) pupil bisecting bifocal lenses (Figs. 3.2 and 6.2) with the near addition just enough to convert ET into esophoria. Measuring the AC/A ratio has been discussed in the Text Box 3.1 [2–5].

3. Non-refractive hypoaccommodative ET presents as ET for near fixation due to increased accommodative effort to overcome a weakness of accommodation (remote near point of accommodation). This entity is seldom seen, and both bifocals and medial rectus weakening procedures are recommended for its management [6].

4. Partially accommodative ET is diagnosed when only a part of the deviation is due to accommodative factors (Fig. 3.3). The nonaccommodative component may be congenital or may develop after correction of refractive error [1]. Surgery is indicated to correct only the static deviation after refractive correction.

3.2.2 Nonaccommodative ET

The distinctive feature between accommodative and nonaccommodative esotropia is the absence of disparity in deviation while fixating upon a near or distant target. The following are the common subtypes of nonaccommodative esotropia:

Text Box 3.1: Measuring the AC/A Ratio

The AC/A ratio can be measured either by the gradient method or the hetero-phoria method. The gradient method gives a better estimate of the ratio [2]. The unit for AC/A ratio is prism diopter (Δ)/diopter (D). The ratio in normal subjects varies from about 1.5:1 to 5.5:1 depending on the method used for its calculation and probably also on the race [3–5].

Gradient method

$$AC/A = \frac{N-L}{3}$$

N = Deviation in Δ with proper correction at 33 cm
L = Deviation with addition of +3D lenses at 33 cm to relax accommodation

Heterophoria method

$$AC/A = IPD + \frac{N-D}{3}$$

IPD = Interpupillary distance (in cm)
N = Near deviation (33 cm) in Δ
D = Distance deviation (6 m) in Δ

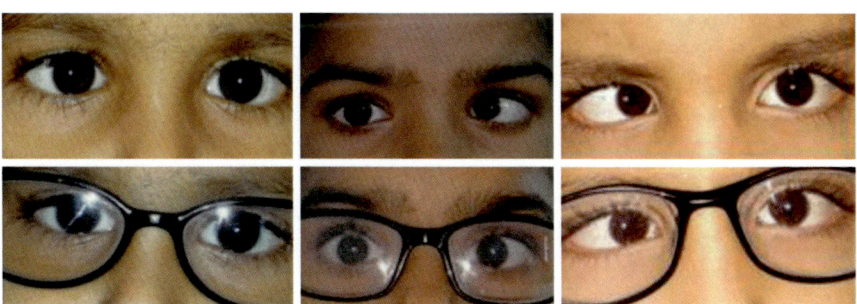

Fig. 3.3 (L to R) Refractive accommodative ET, partially accommodative ET and nonaccommodative (basic type) ET

1. *Essential infantile ET* as the name suggests has an onset in the first year of life and has an unknown aetiology (Fig. 3.4). It is a commonly seen variant and is characterised by a stable, large-angle deviation with asymmetrical optokinetic nystagmus. Amblyopia, crossed fixation and other motility abnormalities like up shoot or down shoot on adduction are frequently associated. It's management is surgical alignment. Surgery should be performed as soon as a fair estimate of the

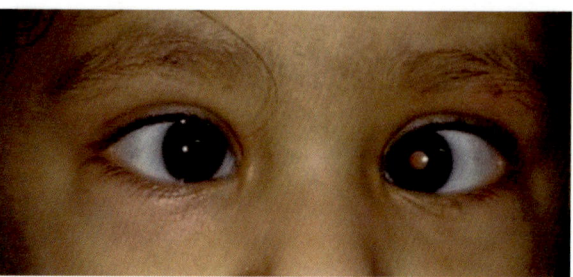

Fig. 3.4 Infantile ET

Text Box 3.2: Choice of Surgery in Infantile ET

Children below 6 years	Bimedial recession
Patients with demonstrable binocularity	Bimedial recession
Patients with no binocular functions	MR Recession + LR Resection of non-dominant eye
Children unwilling/unfit for surgery	Inj. botulinum toxin in both medial recti

amount of deviation can be made. The surgery recommended is bimedial recession in children and medial rectus recession with lateral rectus resection of the non-dominant eye in patients with poor prognosis for recovery of binocularity (Text Box 3.2). For children in whom early surgery is not possible, botulinum toxin may be considered as an alternative (Chap. 8). Frequently, multiple surgeries are required and binocular functions remain subnormal in long term. Postoperative rehabilitation should be aimed towards amblyopia management.

2. *Acquired or basic ET* has a gradual onset after infancy with no disparity between near and distance deviation. Amblyopia management should be followed by surgical alignment.

3. *Acute onset comitant ET* should be carefully differentiated from paralytic strabismus paying careful attention to motility limitation (Chap. 1). This entity should be managed by specialists.

4. *Convergence excess ET* occurs due to excessive convergence in the presence of normal accommodation. Large bilateral MR recession or posterior fixation sutures (Faden's procedure) on them may be indicated for treatment [1].

3.2.3 Sensory ET

Sensory ET occurs secondary to poor vision in one eye. Treatment consists of correcting the underlying cause of poor vision and amblyopia therapy if the cause is treatable. Alignment should be considered even for blind eyes as the psychosocial impact of cosmetic disfigurement is significant [7–9].

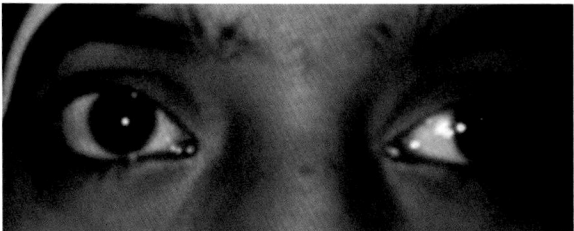

Fig. 3.5 Exotropia left eye

3.2.4 Microtropia

Microtropia is a small-angle (lesser than 5°) ET associated with abnormal retinal correspondence, amblyopia, normal peripheral fusion and defective stereopsis. It is usually diagnosed in older children and adults, in whom it does not require treatment.

3.2.5 ET with Neurological Abnormalities

Children with neurological abnormalities like cerebral palsy often have associated strabismus, most frequently ET [10]. This may present in infancy or later and may show large variability over time. Considering the variability and high risk for general anaesthesia, we manage these children by amblyopia prevention therapy and botulinum toxin initially. Surgical management has a satisfactory outcome in about 50% of children [11].

3.3 Exotropia

Unlike ET, which present as a conglomerate of discreet underlying pathologies, exodeviations are more uniform in their presentation. Exophoria X, intermittent exotropia X (T) and constant exotropia XT may usually be considered as continuum of the same spectrum with progressively worsening fusional reserves [12]. The onset is in early childhood, but usually the patients present as adults when the amplitude of accommodation and tonic convergence begin to decline. As decompensation of exophoria begins, the patient may complain of diplopia, asthenopia or photophobia (due to absence of near clues which help in control the deviation). As the deviation becomes constant, suppression develops, and patient becomes asymptomatic except for cosmetic disfigurement (Fig. 3.5).

It should be understood that many patients have variability of fusional control depending on alertness, general health, anxiety and willingness to cooperate for examination. It could vary at different time of the day and from one examination to the next. Calhounz et al. have classified XT into IV phases based on the fusional control where a patient in phase I has X at distance only, in phase II has X(T) for distance, phase III has XT for distance and X(T)' for near, and phase IV has constant XT. A phase I patient would be asymptomatic, and there would be a progressive worsening of binocular functions from phase II till phase IV where they would be largely absent (Text Box 3.3).

Text Box 3.3: Phenomenon of Panoramic Vision
Horizontal enlargement of the visual field during binocular viewing is sometimes seen in large angle constant XT. There is absence of any retinal correspondence and the two eyes function independently like in lower species. These individuals enjoy a large horizontal visual field up to 250° at the cost of the binocular vision.

Clinical Tip
Care should be taken to neutralise any effect of fusion mechanisms while evaluating the angle of deviation. Maximum static deviation should be assessed while planning surgical management.

3.3.1 Exotropia Classification

For management it would be also useful to classify XT into the following types

1. *Divergence excess*—when the deviation for distance fixation is at least 15$^\Delta$ (prism dioptres) larger than for near
2. *Convergence insufficiency*—when the deviation for near fixation is at least 15$^\Delta$ larger than for distance
3. *Basic*—when the near and distance deviations are equal or their difference is lesser than 15$^\Delta$
4. *Simulated divergence excess*—which on initial testing has a significantly larger deviation for distance fixation but on elimination of dynamic factors (by occlusion of either eye for 1 h) the near deviation becomes equal to or larger than the distance deviation. This phenomenon is called *convergence after effect*. For this reason all patients with divergence excess type of deviation should undergo an occlusion test by occluding either eye for 1 h [13]. Before removing the patch for measurements (by prism and cover test), the fellow eye should be occluded to prevent even a momentary binocular stimulation that could make the patient control the near deviation.

3.3.2 Exotropia Management

As with all types of strabismus, refractive correction should be the first step in management. Although it is believed that uncorrected myopia plays a role in development to exodeviation by constant under stimulation of convergence [14], this factor has a much lesser importance than hypermetropia in causation of esotropia [11]. Myopia should be fully or slightly overcorrected and least possible hypermetropic correction should be titrated individually to make the patient comfortable. Contact lenses and refractive surgery are known to have a beneficial effect on ocular deviation and may be tried in suitable patients as discussed in Chap. 6 [15, 16].

As in accommodative ET, it has also been suggested to measure the deviation for near fixation through +3.0 D sphere to eliminate the need for accommodation and unmask substantially larger deviation in patients with increased AC/A ratio [17]. This exercise, however, has a very limited role in management planning of XT [11, 18]. Stereoacuity assessment for near and distance should routinely be done in patients with X(T). A progressive deterioration can be an indicator for early surgical intervention.

Role of prisms and orthoptics is limited to improving binocular vision, amblyopia treatment and treating obvious convergence insufficiency. Definite treatment of symptomatic X, X(T) and XT is surgical [11].

Surgery for constant deviations should be performed once the diagnosis is made and reliable measurements made. Surgery is not performed for deviations lesser than 15^{Δ}.

Text Box 3.4: Timing of Surgery in X(T)
Surgery in intermittent exotropia [11, 15–17] should be considered when

- There is progression as evident by:
  - Increased frequency of manifest deviation (>50% of waking hours)
  - Increase in size of basic deviation
  - Evidence of deterioration of distance stereoacuity or development of suppression
- Newcastle control score (NCS) is ≥3/7

NCS is calculated by scoring home and clinic control and totalling the scores (0 being best control and 7 being worst).
Home control is scored 0, 1, 2 or 3 depending on whether the deviation is never noticed, noticed <50% of the time for distance, >50% of the time for distance or seen for both near and distance.
Clinic control is scored (*separately* for distance and near) 0, 1 or 2 depending on whether the deviation is manifest only after cover test with spontaneous control or control occurs after a blink or gets manifest spontaneously.

Timing of surgery for X(T) is decided according to information in Text Box 3.4 [11, 19–21]. Choice of surgery is summarised in the Text Box 3.5 [11]. Botulinum toxin injection has also been suggested for management in children and adults [22, 23].

Short- to medium-term results of exotropia surgery are good with majority of patients achieving reduction in static angle and developing better control of deviation. The latter can be attributed to better sensory status in most XT patients compared to ET. However, long-term prognosis is guarded as recurrences are common.

Sensory XT occurs secondary to poor vision in one eye. Alignment is recommended for cosmesis and associated psychosocial benefits [6, 7].

Text Box 3.5: Choice of Surgery in XT according to types

Divergence excess	Bilateral LR recession
Convergence insufficiency	1. Bimedial resection (if deviation present only for near)
	2. LR recession + MR resection of 1 eye
Basic type and simulated divergence excess	LR recession + MR resection of non-dominant eye
Sensory XT	LR recession + MR resection of blind eye

3.4 Summary

- Horizontal comitant strabismus forms the commonest group of strabismus and can be broadly classified into esotropia and exotropia.
- Primary anomaly is believed to lie in the higher centres. Dynamic factors may be superimposed making the management challenging.
- Prescribing appropriate refractive correction is the essential first step in management.
- Deviation should always be measured for near and distance. Any change in deviation with refractive correction must also be noted.
- Early surgery is indicated in essential infantile esotropia.
- Exotropia may be considered a clinical spectrum with exophoria and constant exotropia as the two extremes, indicating a progressive loss of fusional reserves.
- While assessing exotropia, all efforts must be made to unmask the maximum deviation before planning surgical correction.
- X(T) is common; surgical intervention may be indicated in the presence of worsening stereoacuity.
- Surgery is considered only for the static component of deviation with the aim to restore stable fusion at near and distance fixation.

3.5 Multiple Choice Questions

1. Infantile esotropia is characterised by all of the following *except*:
   (a) Large-angle deviation
   (b) Cross fixation
   (c) Inferior oblique overaction
   (d) High hypermetropia

Answer: (d) Infantile esotropia is usually not associated with significant refractive error.

2. True about management of intermittent exotropia X(T)
   (a) When the exotropia occurs during more than 50% of waking hours, surgery should be performed.
   (b) If diplopia vanishes in a patient who previously had diplopia, it is a good prognostic sign.
   (c) Near stereoacuity is more important than distant stereoacuity as it worsens earlier.
   (d) All of the above.

Answer: (a) Exotropia occurring for more than 50% of waking hours is indication of surgery. If diplopia vanishes in a patient of X(T), it is a bad sign as it signifies suppression. Distance stereoacuity deteriorates first in X(T).

3. Which of the following best defines accommodative esotropias?
   (a) Onset at 3–4 years of age with deviation equal for near and distance.
   (b) Onset at 2–3 years of age, deviation for near more than distance, may be associated with hypermetropia or high AC/A ratio.
   (c) Onset <1 year of age and high AC/A ratio.
   (d) Onset at 2–3 years of age, deviation for distance more than near.

Answer: (b) Accommodative ET is caused by increased accommodative effort (due to hypermetropia) or an abnormally high AC/A ratio. Its onset is usually between 2 and 3 years of age, and the deviation for near fixation is larger than that for distance.

4. 1 mm decentration of corneal reflex corresponds to:
   (a) 5°
   (b) 7°
   (c) 5.5°
   (d) 6°

Answer: (b) 1 mm decentration of corneal reflection corresponds to 7° of deviation in visual axis.

References

1. von Noorden GK, Campos EC. Chapter 16: Esodeviations. In: Binocular vision and ocular motility. 6th ed. St. Louis: Mosby; 2002. p. 311–49.
2. Ogle KN, Martens TG, Dyer JA. Oculomotor imbalance in binocular vision and fixation disparity. Philadelphia: Lea & Febiger; 1967.
3. Murray C, Newsham D. Normative values for the accommodative convergence to accommodation ratio (AC/A). Invest Ophthalmol Vis Sci. 2010;51:801.

4. Jackson JH, Arnoldi K. The gradient AC/A ratio: what's really normal? Am Orthopt J. 2004;54:125–32.
5. Sen DK, Malik S. Accommodative-convergence over accommodation (AC/A) ratio (in normal Indian subjects). Indian J Ophthalmol. 1972;20:153–7.
6. Vivian AJ, Lyons CJ, Burke J. Controversy in the management of convergence excess esotropia. Br J Ophthalmol. 2002;86(8):923–9.
7. Durnian JM, Noonan CP, Marsh IB. The psychosocial effects of adult strabismus: a review. Br J Ophthalmol. 2011;95:450–3.
8. Olitsky SE, Sudesh S, Graziano A, Hamblen J, Brooks SE, Shaha SH. The negative psychosocial impact of strabismus in adults. J AAPOS. 1999;3(4):209–11.
9. Mojon-Azzi SM, Kunz A, Mojon DS. Strabismus and discrimination in children: are children with strabismus invited to fewer birthday parties? Br J Ophthalmol. 2011;95:473–6.
10. Collins ML. Strabismus in cerebral palsy: when and why to operate. Am Orthopt J. 2014;64:17–20.
11. Ghasia F, Brunstrom-Hernandez J, Tychsen L. Repair of strabismus and binocular fusion in children with cerebral palsy: gross motor function classification scale. Invest Ophthalmol Vis Sci. 2011;52(10):7664–71.
12. von Noorden GK, Campos EC. Chapter 17: Exodeviations. In: Binocular vision and ocular motility. 6th ed. St. Louis: Mosby; 2002. p. 356–76.
13. Wright KW, Spiegel PH, Thompson LS. Chapter 8: Exotropia. In: Handbook of pediatric strabismus and amblyopia. New York: Springer; 2006. p. 270–1.
14. Donders FC. An essay on the nature and the consequences of anomalies of refraction, Oliver CA, editor. Philadelphia: P Blakiston's Son & Co; 1899. p. 59.
15. Herman JS, Johnson R. The accommodation requirement in myopia. A comparison of contact lens and spectacles. Arch Ophthalmol. 1966;76:47–51.
16. Agrawal S, Singh V, Yadav A, Katiyar V. Orthoptic relevance of refractive correction in the phakic plane in unilateral high refractive errors in adults. Oman J Ophthalmol. 2016;9:196–8.
17. Brown HW. Discussion of paper by Burian HM, Franceschetti AT: Evaluation of diagnostic methods for the classification of exodeviations. Trans Am Ophthalmol Soc. 1970;68:56.
18. Burian HM, Franceschetti AT. Evaluation of diagnostic methods for classification of exodeviations. Trans Am Ophthalmol Soc. 1970;68:56.
19. Haggerty H, et al. The Newcastle Control Score: a new method of grading the severity of intermittent distance exotropia. Br J Ophthalmol. 2004;88:233–5.
20. Baker JD, Schweers M, Petrunak J. Is earlier surgery a sensory benefit in treatment of intermittent exotropia? In: Lennerstrand G, editor. Advances in strabismology, Proceedings of the eighth Meeting of the International Strabismological Association, Maatricht, Dept 10–12, 1988. Buren, The Netherlands: Aeolus Press; 1999. p. 289.
21. Kelkar JA, Gopal S, Shah RB, Kelkar AS. Intermittent exotropia: surgical treatment strategies. Indian J Ophthalmol. 2015;63:566–9.
22. Spencer RF, Tucker MG, Choi RY, McNeer KW. Botulinum toxin management of childhood intermittent exotropia. Ophthalmology. 1997;104(11):1762–7.
23. Etezad Razavi M, Sharifi M, Armanfar F. Efficacy of botulinum toxin in the treatment of intermittent exotropia. Strabismus. 2014;22(4):176–81.

Incomitant Strabismus and Principles of Its Management

4

Chong-Bin Tsai and Rajat M. Srivastava

4.1 Introduction

Differentiation between comitant and incomitant strabismus is an important task for the general ophthalmologist managing strabismus. The paralyses or restrictions underlying incomitant strabismus may imply potentially dangerous disorders that should be treated promptly. Early detection and proper management are necessary to achieve good clinical outcome.

4.2 Basics of Incomitant Strabismus

We initially discuss some concepts related to the understanding of incomitant strabismus. Few of these have already been dealt with in the earlier chapters but are mentioned here to make the understanding clearer.

4.2.1 Comitance and Incomitance

The word "comitant" was originated from the word "concomitant." Concomitant is defined as "accompanying especially in a subordinate or incidental way" in Merriam-Webster Dictionary. It implies that, despite of the strabismic deviation,

C.-B. Tsai (✉)
Department of Ophthalmology, Chiayi Christian Hospital, Chiayi City, Taiwan

Department of Hospital and Health Care Administration, Chia Nan University of Pharmacy and Science, Chiayi, Taiwan

R. M. Srivastava
Department of Ophthalmology, King George's Medical University, Lucknow, India

© Springer Nature Singapore Pte Ltd. 2019
S. Agrawal (ed.), *Strabismus*, https://doi.org/10.1007/978-981-13-1126-0_4

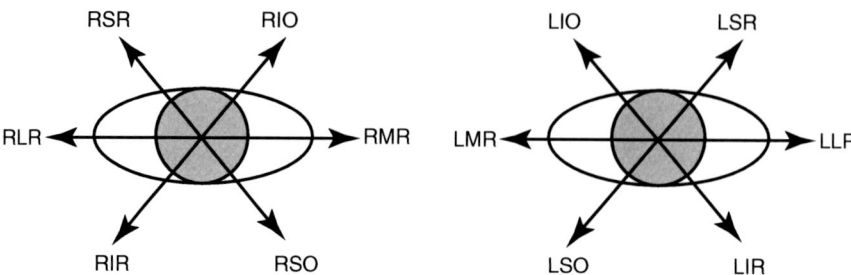

Fig. 4.1 Yoke muscles in six cardinal directions of gaze

one eye accompanies the other eye in all direction of gaze. Duane proposed the briefer term "comitant," which is now universally accepted in the literatures [1].

In a comitant strabismus, the amount of deviation remains the same in all direction of gaze. To maintain the comitance, the Hering's law of equal innervation, also called the law of motor correspondence, plays a major role [2]. According to this, the yoke muscles in each eye receive equal impulses to contract together to move the eyes toward the desired direction (Fig. 4.1). This comitance can be disturbed by many factors, which results in incomitant (noncomitant) strabismus. In an incomitant strabismus, the amount of deviation varies in different directions of gaze. Clinically, most incomitant strabismus are paralytic, restrictive, or of combined mechanism. Factors causing incomitance can be related to abnormalities of the extraocular muscles, orbit, neuromuscular junction, cranial nerves or their nuclei, supranuclear control, or combined mechanisms.

4.2.2   Primary Deviation and Secondary Deviation

A characteristic of incomitant strabismus is that the deviation varies with different fixating eye. The examiner measures the deviation, as is discussed in Chap. 2. It is to be remembered that the prism is not placed over the fixating eye. Using the measurement of exotropia as an example, when the examiner holds a base-in prism over the right eye, the right eye will be viewing in an abducted position as it looks through the prism. The left eye remains in its primary position during the measurement. Therefore, the left eye is the fixating eye during the measurement.

When the non-paretic or nonrestricted eye is used to fixate, the deviation measured is the primary deviation (measurement done with prisms over the primarily squinting eye). When the paretic or restricted eye is used to fixate (prisms over the normal eye), the deviation measured is the secondary deviation. In the condition of paralysis or restriction, the affected eye will need increased innervation to the paralyzed muscle to move to the fixating position. According to Hering's law, the increased amount of innervation will flow to the yoke muscle in the fellow eye, and this extra innervation will cause its excessive contraction exaggerating the strength disparity between these two yoke muscles. The result is an increased deviation when the affected eye is used for fixating. This is the reason why *the secondary deviation is always greater than the primary deviation*.

4.2.3   Spread of Comitance

The difference in primary and secondary deviation is most obvious when the paresis is recent. In long-standing paresis of one muscle, changes occur in other extraocular muscles, called "muscle sequelae." The development of muscle sequelae consists the following stages:

1. Overaction of its contralateral agonist (yoke muscle)
2. Overaction of the ipsilateral antagonist
3. Secondary underaction of the antagonist of yoke muscle

For example (Fig. 4.2), in a patient with a right lateral rectus paralysis, an esodeviation will occur which is largest in right gaze (dextroversion). According to Hering's law, the increased amount of innervation necessary to move the paretic right lateral rectus also flows to the left medial rectus (the contralateral agonist) and results in an overaction of left medial rectus. The right medial rectus (the ipsilateral antagonist) is acting unopposed and will be more or less overacting. However, according to Sherrington's law, the right medial rectus is actually receiving lesser inhibitional innervation than normal, and consequently lesser force is required to overcome the right lateral rectus (which is paralyzed) to fixate on a target. Then, according to Hering's law again, the innervation to left lateral rectus (the contralateral antagonist) will also be reduced. The left lateral rectus will be acting like a paralyzed muscle. This phenomenon is called "inhibitional palsy of the contralateral antagonist.". The esodeviation in left gaze (levoversion) would increase and match that in right gaze gradually. The difference between primary and secondary deviation would decrease, and the strabismus becomes concomitant, called "spread of comitance." This development of muscle sequelae occurs more often when the paralysis is long-standing and affects a strongly dominant fixating eye. This phenomenon often makes identification of the primary paretic eye difficult.

4.3   Clinical Approach to Incomitant Strabismus

It is crucial to differentiate paretic or restrictive strabismus from comitant forms of strabismus, not only because the principles of the management of incomitant strabismus are different from that of comitant strabismus, but also because an acquired paretic strabismus may be an initial sign of a sinister neurological abnormality.

When a paralytic strabismus is suspected clinically, the clinician needs to determine the possible underlying etiology. The causes may range from a rather benign microvascular event to a potentially dangerous intracranial lesion. The aim of clinical investigations is to identify the etiology and initiate timely intervention, if required.

The differentiation between acquired and congenital paralyses is essential. In recently acquired paralyses, patients often have symptoms of diplopia, or blurred vision, and are aware of change in head posture. While in congenital paralyses, patients usually adapt to their visual disorder, perhaps with development of suppression. Old photographs are helpful to clarify the time of onset of abnormal head

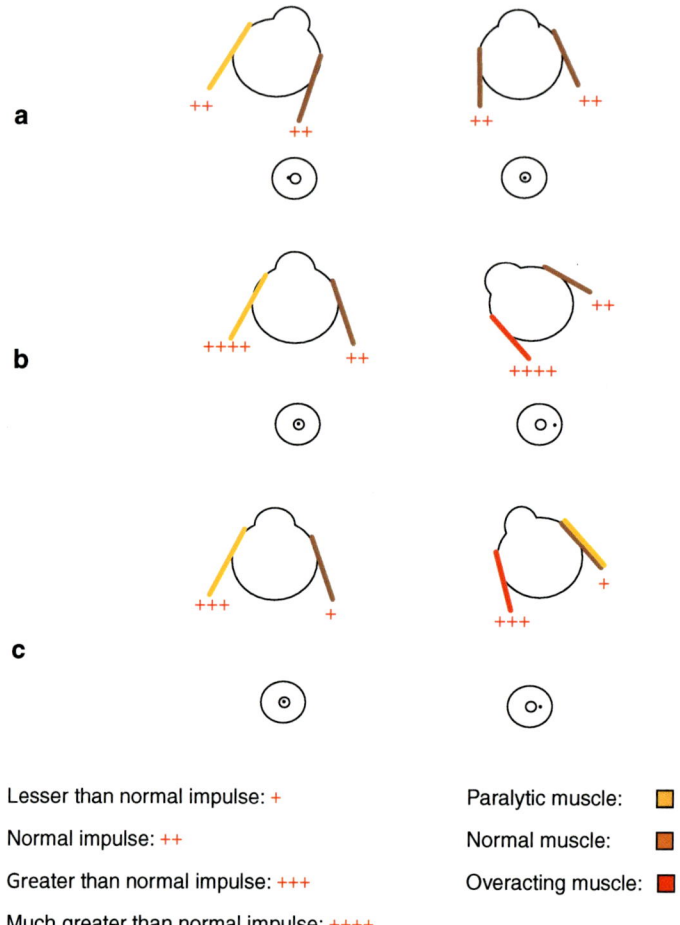

Lesser than normal impulse: +   Paralytic muscle: ■

Normal impulse: ++   Normal muscle: ■

Greater than normal impulse: +++   Overacting muscle: ■

Much greater than normal impulse: ++++

Fig. 4.2 Diagrammatic representation (in the presence of right lateral rectus (RLR) palsy) of the concepts of (a) *primary deviation* in the right eye (RE) which develops esotropia (ET) when normal impulse to contract (++) is reaching all muscles. (b) *Secondary deviation* in left eye (LE) when RE is forced to fixate with a much greater than normal impulse to contract (++++) reaching the paralyzed RLR and its yoke muscle, the left medial rectus (LMR). The normal LMR causes a much larger deviation in LE. (c) *Inhibitional palsy* of left lateral rectus (LLR) develops over time if the RE is dominant and prefers to fixate. The antagonist of the paralyzed muscle, i.e., RMR, starts receiving lesser impulse to contract as it is acting against a muscle (RLR) with reduced tonus. The same reduced impulse gets transmitted to the yoke of the antagonist of the paralyzed muscle, i.e., the LLR which starts underacting. Note that the secondary deviation reduces, compared to (b)

posture. Detailed history of antecedent events, including trauma, viral infection, meningitis, and microvascular risk factors such as diabetes mellitus, hypertension, and hyperlipidemia are important clues to potential causes.

The decision of whether to order neuroimaging in acquired paralyses is challenging to clinicians. In an era with many advances in treatment of stroke, neoplasm and demyelinating diseases, early diagnosis of these conditions provides better clinical outcomes [3]. Multiple cranial nerve involvement and associated neurological symptoms and signs, such as headache, papilledema, and seizures, are indications for prompt neuroimaging. In isolated acquired ocular motor neuropathies, age of presentation and the cranial nerve involved are important factors for decision-making. Acute presentation in children almost always warrants a neuroimaging.

4.3.1 History Taking

The assessment starts with focused history taking as discussed in Chap. 2. The following information should be collected.

- The age of onset of the deviation. The circumstance under which the deviation becomes worse. Is it constant or intermittent? Is it unilateral or alternating? Is it worse at the end of the day?
- Associated symptoms, including blurred vision, double vision, eye strain, eye pain, watering, closing one eye in bright light, anomalous head posture, headache, dizziness, weakness and numbness of face, or extremities.
- Past ocular history, including glasses, patching, previous surgery, or trauma.
- Past history, including prematurity, developmental delay, hearing impairment, diabetes mellitus, hypertension, hyperlipidemia, trauma, or other systemic or neurological disorders.
- Family history, including ocular and systemic history, especially hereditary disorders.

Infants often have variable ocular deviation in the first month of life (oculomotor instability of infancy) [4]. The deviation of strabismus is nonstable until ~3 months of age. Infantile esotropia often occurs by 6 months of age. Accommodative esotropia typically occurs between 2 and 3 years of age. The age of onset for intermittent exotropia varies but is usually between 6 months and 4 years of age [5].

4.3.2 Head Posture

Anomalous head posture (AHP), compensatory head posture (CHP), or torticollis can result from ocular or non-ocular causes. Ocular AHP is often a compensatory response to minimize diplopia and improve the field of binocular vision in strabismus. The presence of AHP in a strabismus patient is suggestive of binocularity, and patching of one eye should eliminate it. In infantile nystagmus syndrome, AHP has been assumed to extend the foveation period and to adapt to the position of a strong dominant eye (Fig. 4.3) [6]. AHPs can be observed at any age, even as early as 6 months of age, when an infant just starts to sit unsupported. Prolonged AHP in children often results in facial asymmetry and influences musculoskeletal developments and should thus be corrected as early as possible.

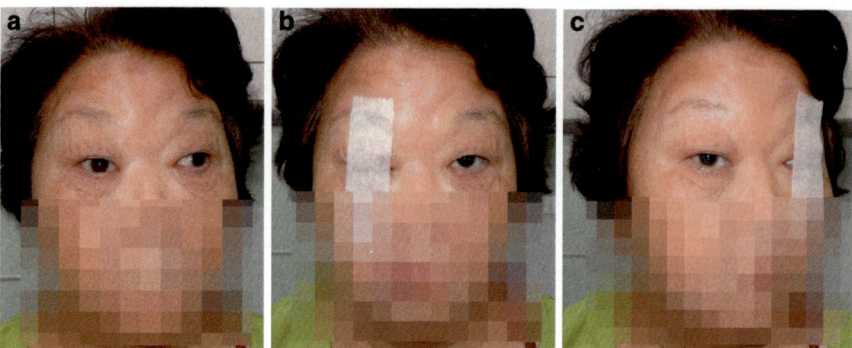

Fig. 4.3 Anomalous head posture (AHP) in a patient with congenital nystagmus with left exotropia (LXT) (**a**). The AHP is because of the fixating right eye (RE) occlusion of which eliminates the AHP (**b**); however, occlusion of the non-fixating left eye (LE) has no effect on it (**c**) (Note: This example should be considered as an exception rather than rule as in most patients with strabismus, AHP corrects with occlusion of either eye)

AHP has three components: (a) face turn, (b) head tilt, and (c) chin elevation or depression (Fig. 1.9). The axis of AHP is helpful in the diagnosis. A face turn may be associated with sixth nerve palsy (to the affected side), Brown syndrome (to the unaffected side), Duane syndrome, or homonymous hemianopia. A head tilt may be associated with superior oblique palsy (to the unaffected side), dissociated vertical deviation, or torsional nystagmus. A chin up/down may be associated with A and V patterns, thyroid eye disease, ptosis, Brown syndrome (chin up), or congenital cranial dysinnervation disorders. Patients with infantile nystagmus syndrome may have combined forms of AHP that include face turn, head tilt, and chin up/down to take advantage of the horizontal, torsional, and vertical components of their null points.

4.3.3 Ocular Movements

Ductions are monocular eye movements. Versions are conjugate binocular eye movements. To measure ductions, the examiner covers one of the patient's eyes and asks the patient to follow a fixation target with the other eye. To measure versions, the patients are examined with both eyes uncovered. In general, ductions are slightly greater than versions. If versions are normal, ductions are usually normal (see Chap. 1 also).

The examiner can follow a useful guideline to judge normal abduction and adduction. In full adduction, the nasal third of cornea is at the position of lower lacrimal punctum. In full abduction, the temporal corneal limbus touches the lateral canthus. Underactions are graded on a scale of 0 to −4, in which 0 indicates full ductions and −4 indicates no movement beyond the primary position. If the eye cannot even reach the primary position, a scale of −5 is recorded (Fig. 4.4).

Right eye in an attempted abduction

Graded on a scale of 0 to –5

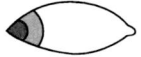

0 indicates that 100% of movement remains

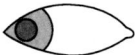

–1 indicates that 75% of movement remains

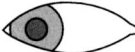

–2 indicates that 50% of movement remains

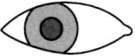

–3 indicates that 25% of movement remains

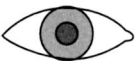

–4 indicates that no movement beyond the midline

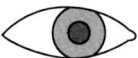

–5 indicates that the eye cannot not reach the midline

Right eye in an attempted adduction

Graded on a scale of 0 to –5

0 indicates that 100% of movement remains

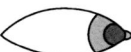

–1 indicates that 75% of movement remains

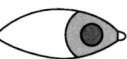

–2 indicates that 50% of movement remains

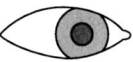

–3 indicates that 25% of movement remains

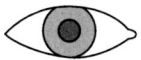

–4 indicates that no movement beyond the midline

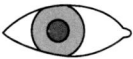

–5 indicates that the eye cannot not reach the midline

Fig. 4.4 Documentation of ocular ductions

Vertical ocular rotations are more complex as the vertical muscles have different secondary and tertiary actions as the globe rotates. However, an asymmetry of elevation (supraduction) straight upward or depression (infraduction) straight downward indicates possible muscle paresis or restriction. In full elevation, the lower limbus of cornea can pass above an imaginary horizontal line through lateral canthus. In full depression, the upper limbus of cornea can easily pass several millimeters below an imaginary horizontal line through lateral canthus, and the pupil gets covered by the lower lid. It is useful to record the limitation in ocular movements by photographs of the patient (Chap. 1).

When limitation of ductions is observed, it is necessary to perform *forced duction test* (FDT) to differentiate restriction from paresis. Office forced duction testing can usually be performed successfully in cooperative adults. The conjunctiva is anesthetized with topical 0.5% proparacaine eyedrops. An eyelid speculum is applied. The non-testing eye is covered. The patient is instructed to look as far as possible in the direction of suspected limited duction. The examiner grasps the conjunctiva near limbus with fixation forceps and tries to rotate the globe further in the direction of limited duction. If the globe cannot be passively rotated further, restriction is present, and the result is recorded as positive. If further rotation is possible, the result is negative, and paresis may be the cause of the limited duction. FDT and force generation test (FGT) are discussed in Chap. 6.

The overaction of inferior oblique is often assessed during examination for versions. Overaction of the adducting eye is assessed, and the other eye (abducting eye) should be fixating during assessment. It should keep looking straight across the lateral canthus. The overaction is graded on a scale of +1 to +4, in which +4 indicates the corneal reflection is located at the lower limbus and +2 indicates the reflection located at midway between the pupil center and lower limbus.

4.3.4   Three-Step Test

In patients with vertical deviation in primary position, the three-step test is a helpful diagnostic algorithm to detect an isolated cyclovertical muscle palsy [7]. The results of this test may be invalid in multiple muscle paralyses, restrictive strabismus, dissociated vertical deviation, and underlying vestibular or supranuclear disease [8]. The test should not be attempted in patients with cervical spine instability.

The examiner determines (a) which eye is hypertrophic in primary position, (b) whether the deviation increases in dextroversion or levoversion, and (c) whether the deviation increases with right or left head tilt. It is useful if the examiner can identify the eye with primary deviation (eye with muscle paralysis) initially.

4.3.4.1 Step 1
The examiner measures the deviation at primary position and marks the suspected underacting muscle groups. For example (Fig. 4.5), if right hypertropia (or left hypotropia) is present at primary position, the suspected underacting muscle groups are inferior rectus and superior oblique of the right eye (RIR and RSO) and superior rectus and left inferior oblique of the left eye (LSR and LIO). If at this stage the paralytic eye can be confirmed by primary and secondary deviation, the suspicion shifts to two muscles only.

4.3.4.2 Step 2
The examiner then determines if the deviation increases in right or left gaze. If the vertical deviation is larger in left gaze, of the four suspected muscles, only two could be underacting in this position, i.e., RSO and LSR. Larger deviation occurs only when the weak muscle is forced to contract due to larger impulse being transmitted to its yoke muscle (Hering's Law). So the suspicion shifts to either RSO or LSR. Also, if the examiner had determined the eye with paralytic muscle earlier, the diagnosis is made at this stage itself.

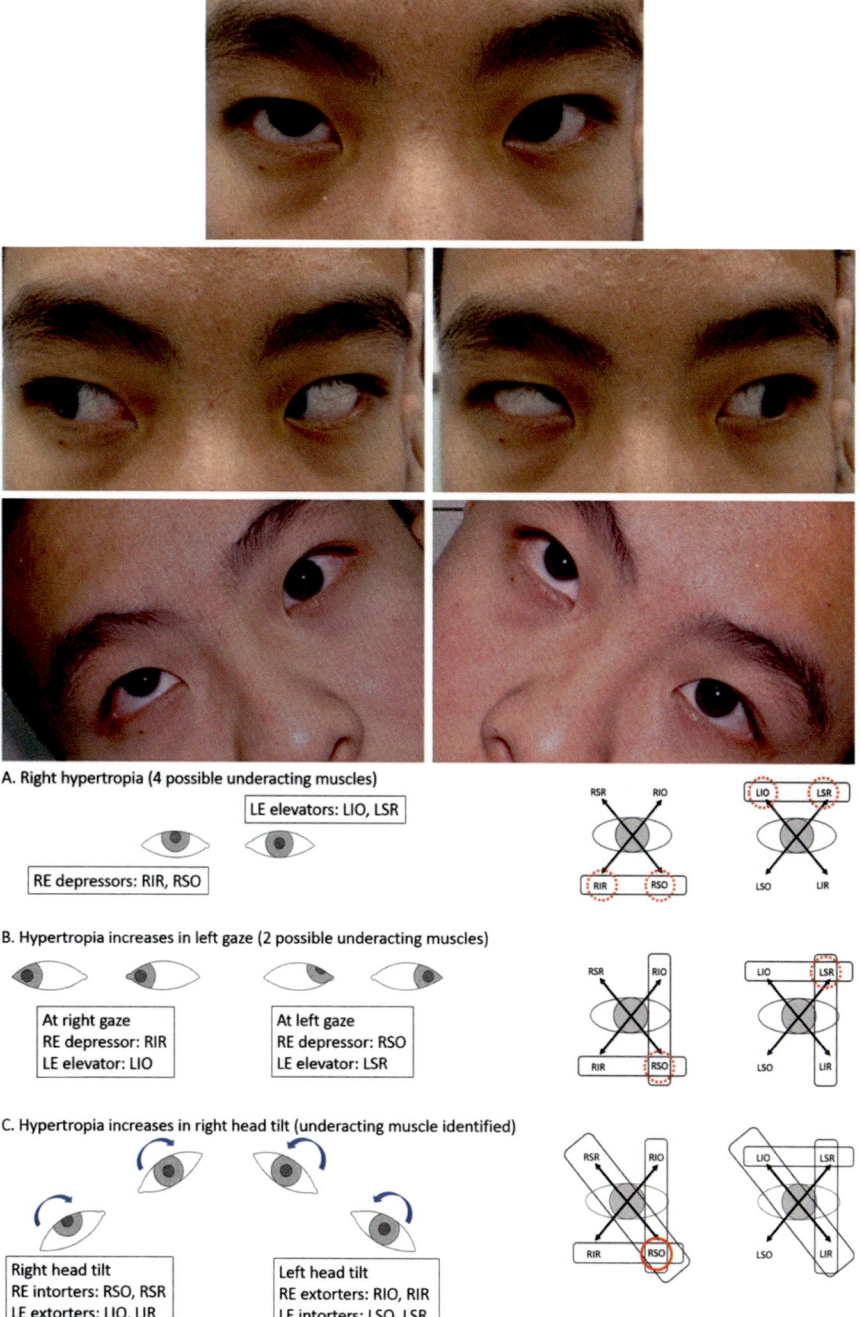

Fig. 4.5 Park's three-step test in right superior oblique palsy

4.3.4.3 Step 3

The examiner performs the Bielschowsky head tilt test by trying to estimate the change in deviation with the patient's head tilted to the right and left. Physiologically, a head tilt will induce compensatory ocular counter roll to reduce the torsions of the eyes relative to space. For instance, a right head tilt will induce incyclotorsion of the right eye and excyclotorsion of the left eye. The two muscles being considered are both intorters (Chap. 1), and right eye intorter (RSO here) would be forced to contract on right head tilt and the left eye intorter (LSR here) on left head tilt. So, if the deviation increases in right head tilt, the paralyzed muscle is RSO.

4.3.5 Hess Chart Test

Hess chart is a valuable tool for investigation of incomitant strabismus. By dissociating the two images of each eye, the test detects the position of fixating eye and non-fixating eye in different directions of gaze. The Hess chart test is a subjective test. It requires good vision in both eyes and foveal projection with normal retinal correspondence.

A standard Hess chart test consists a gray Hess screen with tangential patterns. The cardinal positions of eye movement are shown in red color, operated manually or electrically, sequentially. The patient wears a red and green goggle, with the red filter before the fixating eye. On the Hess screen, there is a central point, which is the primary position, surrounded by an inner field of eight points and outer field of 16 points. The test is performed at a distance of 50 cm. At this test distance, the points on the inner field represent the fixation at 15° from the primary position and the outer field representing the fixation at 30° from the primary position. For subtle underactions or overactions, which are hard to detect by the inner field, the outer field should be examined as the deviation will be more evident as the eye moves further to the field of action of the paralyzed muscle (Fig. 4.6).

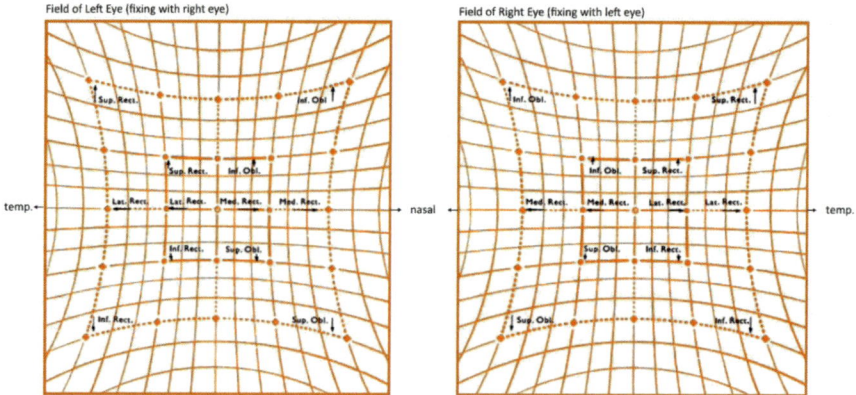

Fig. 4.6 Standard Hess chart

The results are plotted on Hess charts. The charts show deviation field for each eye when non-fixating. The field of left eye is recorded on the left chart and the field of right eye on the right chart. The recorded fields are direct recording of eye deviation. It means that a higher plot indicates a higher eye when the other eye is fixating. The Hess chart records the relative deviation of each eye, that is, a higher recording of one eye should be accompanied by a lower recording of the other eye, perhaps in different amplitude (due to difference in primary and secondary deviations), at the same fixation position.

The interpretation of Hess chart consists three important elements: position, size, and shape. The *position* of the field reflects the position of the eyes. A temporally displaced field reflects an exodeviation, and a nasally displaced field reflects an esodeviation. One should note that the plot of the central point is the deviation in the tested eye when the fixating eye is at the primary position and not the actual position of the tested eye.

The *size* of the field represents the amount of eye movement. An underaction of extraocular muscle will displace the plot interior to the normal field. Therefore, a reduced size indicates a limitation of movement. An overaction of extraocular muscle will displace the plot exterior to the normal field. Therefore, an enlarged size indicates an overacting movement. Comitance is indicated when the size of two field do not differ significantly.

The affected eye usually presents a smaller field. The examiner can identify the primary affected muscle, which shows the greatest underaction, in the eye with a smaller field (the affected eye) if the paresis is recently acquired (Fig. 4.7). The greatest overaction is demonstrated by the contralateral agonist (yoke) of the primary palsied muscle (Fig. 4.8).

Overaction is usually also shown by the ipsilateral antagonist of the primary palsied muscle usually. If the field is reduced at opposite directions, that is, underaction of a primary affected muscle as well as underaction of its ipsilateral antagonist, a mechanical restriction should be considered (Figs. 4.9 and 4.10).

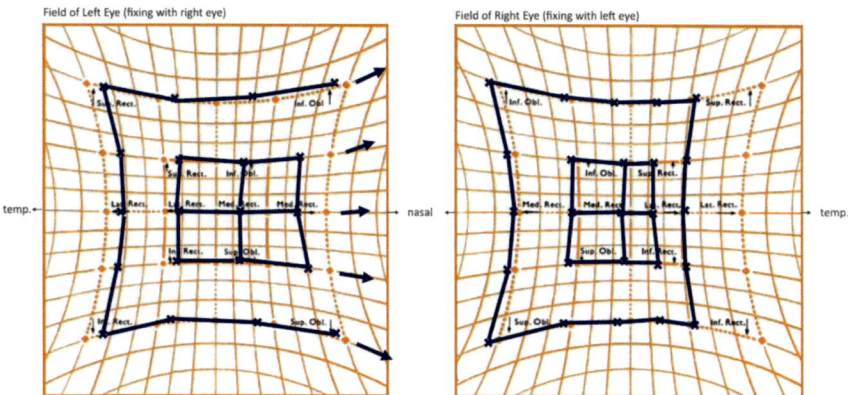

Fig. 4.7 Hess chart of right sixth nerve palsy

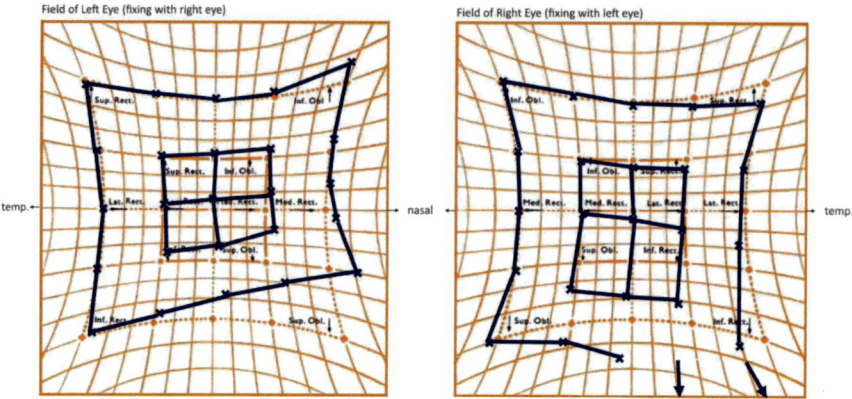

Fig. 4.8 Hess chart of left superior oblique palsy

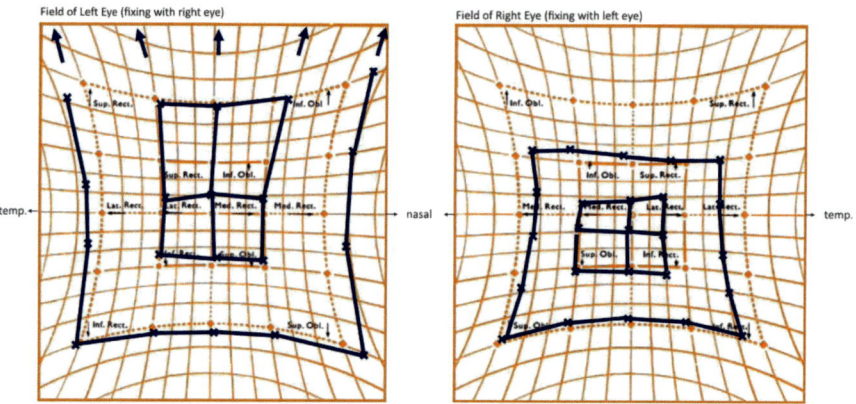

Fig. 4.9 Hess chart of thyroid eye disease with right inferior rectus fibrosis

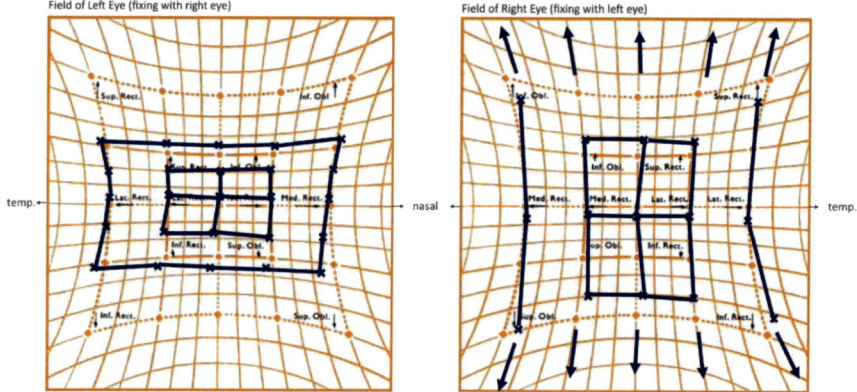

Fig. 4.10 Hess chart of left orbital floor fracture

The *shape* of the field implies the tilting of the field. It occurs when different amount of deviation is measured at different direction of gaze. A-V patterns are the most common examples of tilted shape of field. It should be noted that the tilted field does not indicate torsion.

4.3.6 Diplopia Charting

It is another simple yet effective test to evaluate incomitant strabismus. The test is performed using red and green glasses after eliminating any anomalous head posture of the patient. The details of this test are discussed in Chap. 2. Characteristic diplopia patterns also help in identification of the paralyzed muscle/s.

4.4 Salient Features of Individual Cranial Nerve Palsies

4.4.1 Sixth Nerve Palsy

Sixth nerve palsy is the most common cranial motor nerve palsy (Fig. 4.11). The patients commonly present with complains of sudden onset horizontal diplopia. Clinical findings include presence of face turn to the side of paralysis and esotropia with limitation of abduction in the affected eye. Uncrossed horizontal diplopia is characteristic in this condition. The anatomic position of the sixth cranial nerve makes it vulnerable to lesions from cerebellopontine angle and skull base. Simultaneous involvement of adjacent fifth, seventh, and eighth nerves is common. Neuroimaging is recommended for patients under 50 years of age, especially when multiple cranial nerves are involved. Isolated sixth nerve palsy in patients over 50 years of age with microvascular risk factors is often ischemic and

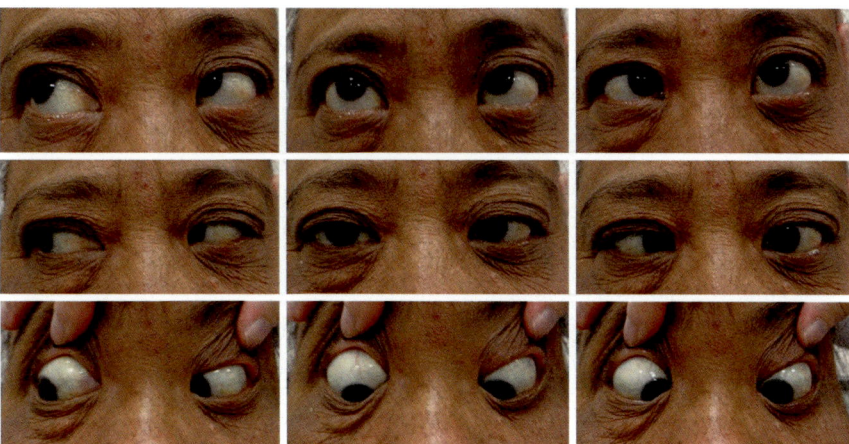

Fig. 4.11 Left sixth nerve palsy

can be followed for 3 months before neuroimaging [9]. Congenital sixth nerve palsy is rare in children. A congenital isolated abduction deficit in children should always raise suspicion of Duane syndrome. Neoplasms are the commonest cause of acquired sixth nerve palsy in children. Neuroimaging is thus recommended (Table 4.1).

4.4.2 Third Nerve Palsy

By virtue of extensive motor innervations of ocular structures, third cranial nerve palsy may have varied presentation. A complete third nerve palsy with pupil involvement typically presents with ptosis and dilated non-reacting pupil with eye in abducted and slightly hypotropic position (Fig. 4.12). A partial third nerve palsy may present with an isolated or multiple extraocular muscle palsy which may or may not involve the pupil. Among the extraocular muscles, isolated inferior oblique palsy is the rarest.

It is crucial to check the pupillary function when evaluating the third nerve palsy. The pupillomotor fibers of third nerve run on the dorsomedial surface of the nerve and are vulnerable to compression by aneurysm arising from posterior communicating artery (PcoA). A pupil involving third nerve palsy, complete or partial, is an indication for emergent neuroimaging to rule out the possibility of aneurysm.

When there is no evidence of pupillary dysfunction (pupil-sparing), the extent of third nerve palsy determines the next step. A pupil-sparing complete third nerve palsy in patients over 50 years of age most likely results from ischemic cranial neuropathy, especially when with the accompanying microvascular risk factors, such as diabetes mellitus, hypertension, or hyperlipidemia, exist. The palsy usually improves within 3–6 months. Neuroimaging is not required, except when the expected recovery does not occur or the palsy progresses or aberrant regeneration occurs in a nontraumatic palsy [21].

However, a pupil-sparing partial third nerve palsy has a different clinical meaning and often warrants imaging. Partial palsy may imply that some fibers of the third nerve are affected by a compressive lesion, and the other fibers, together with pupillomotor fibers, are not affected yet. The palsy may progress and later involve the pupil.

Another sign indicative of an underlying space occupying lesion is primary aberrant regeneration. Commonly, aberrant regeneration occurs after injuries when surviving nerve fibers grow to reinnervate the muscle and their misrouting occurs. However, when aberrant regeneration occurs in absence of trauma (in a presumed microvascular ischemic neuropathy), a compressive lesion should be suspected and neuroimaging should be obtained.

Third nerve palsy in children has different clinical features compared to adults. Commonest etiology is congenital, followed by trauma, viral infections, and tumor (Table 4.1). Aberrant regeneration is common in children. Pupil involvement is common in congenital form and does not suggest a compressive lesion as in adults [22]. Associated neurological anomalies such as arachnoid cyst and optic hypoplasia may exist. Neuroimaging is recommended in all children with third nerve palsy [7].

Table 4.1 Common causes of palsy of ocular motor nerves and indications for neuroimaging

	N III (Oculomotor)		N IV (Trochlear)		N VI (Abducens)	
	Children [7, 10–13]	Adults [14]	Children [15, 16]	Adults [17]	Children [18–20]	Adults [8]
Etiology (in decreasing frequency)	Congenital, trauma, infection, tumor	Aneurysm, microvasculopathy[a], trauma	Congenital, trauma, idiopathic	Congenital, trauma, microvasculopathy[a]	Tumor, hydrocephalus, trauma, infection	Microvasculopathy[a], trauma, tumor
Indications for neuroimaging	All patients	Pupil involvement, below 50 years (not at risk for microvasculopathy), non-resolving till 3 months, trauma, aberrant regeneration in non-traumatic palsy, partial palsy	Trauma	Acquired palsy below 50 years (not at risk for microvasculopathy), non-resolving till 3 months, trauma	All patients	Patients below 50 years (not at risk for microvasculopathy), non-resolving till 3 months, trauma

[a]Common microvasculopathies are diabetes mellitus and hypertension

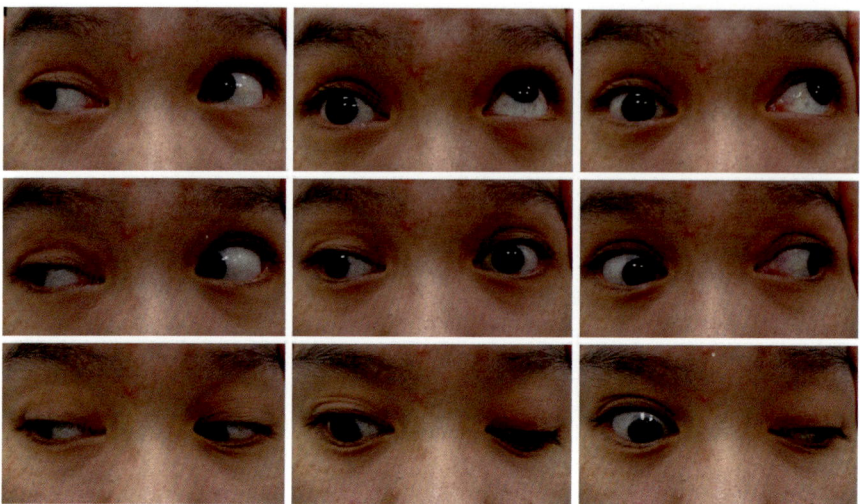

Fig. 4.12 Right third nerve palsy

4.4.3 Fourth Nerve Palsy

Fourth nerve palsies are usually congenital (Table 4.1, Fig. 4.13), and patients may be asymptomatic at early age. There can be associated anomalies of the nerve itself, tendon of superior oblique muscle, structure of trochlea, or insertion site on the globe.

Most of the acquired forms of fourth nerve palsy are caused by trauma or microvascular ischemia. Fourth nerve is the only cranial nerve exiting from dorsal midbrain and has the longest intracranial course. It is therefore vulnerable to closed head trauma. Patients with acquired palsy present with asthenopic symptoms, vertical diplopia, and AHP (head tilt to opposite side of palsy). Patients often complain of troublesome diplopia while climbing down the stairs.

Considering the low yield of neuroimaging in acquired non-traumatic fourth nerve palsies, patients over 50 years of age with microvascular risk factors can usually be followed for 3 months before neuroimaging [23].

4.5 Principles of Nonsurgical Management for Incomitant Strabismus

Nonsurgical management is aimed at preventing complications like amblyopia, contractures, etc. and making the patient comfortable till recovery occurs or definite surgical management is done. The patient is made comfortable by increasing the

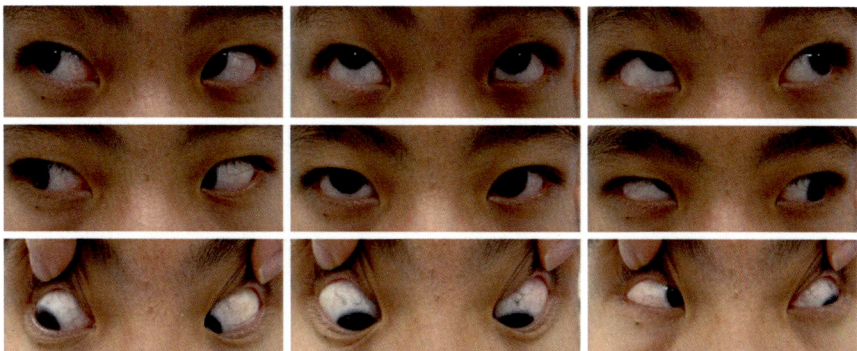

Fig. 4.13 Right fourth nerve paresis. Note the increased right hypertropia in levoversion and reduced motility of right eye in levodepression

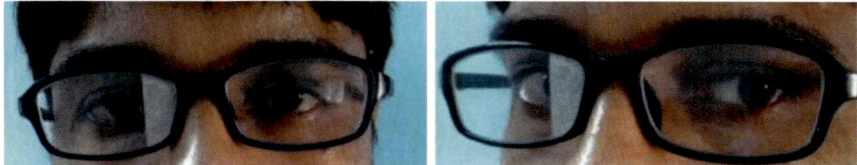

Fig. 4.14 Segmental occlusion for diplopia in levoversion

diplopia-free field, eliminating head posture, and ensuring better cosmesis during the recovery. Nonsurgical options may be considered for long-term management in small-angle deviations specifically when the primary and downgazes are diplopia-free or when the surgery has to be delayed for various reasons. These are discussed in Chap. 5.

Children should be allowed to adopt a head posture as it allows binocular fusion. Alternate occlusion (daily closure of one eye alternately) prevents contractures and eliminates diplopia [17]. It also prevents amblyopia in small children. For small-angle deviations, Fresnel prisms may be tried; however, their utility is limited due to incomitance of deviations. Segmental occlusion of one eye in the direction of diplopia (Fig. 4.14) is also useful in selected cases [24].

In sixth nerve palsy, botulinum toxin is useful in normalization of head posture and increasing the diplopia-free field. It also prevents contractures, improves the patients subjectively, and is believed to reduce the length of morbidity [25–27]. Two to three units are injected in the antagonist or the yoke of the paralyzed muscle. Its utility is limited in third nerve palsy because of multiple extraocular muscle involvement. Botulinum toxin is discussed in Chap. 9.

4.6 Principles of Surgical Management for Incomitant Strabismus

To achieve a good clinical outcome, the surgeon must identify all underlying mechanisms of incomitant strabismus before surgical planning. The mechanisms may be restrictive, paralytic, or combined. Considerations about timing of surgery, procedure, and expected outcome differ for different disease entities. The family must be informed that expecting complete normalization of motility is unrealistic, and the surgery is targeted at restoring binocular single vision in primary and downgazes only.

4.6.1 Paralytic Strabismus

For acquired cranial nerve palsies resulting from trauma, compression or microvascular ischemia surgeries are usually withheld for a recovery period of 6 months after onset or even longer if the recovery is ongoing. In the recovery period, prisms, occlusion, or botulinum toxin are used as discussed in the previous section.

4.6.1.1 Sixth Nerve Palsy

The surgical treatment of sixth nerve palsy depends on the amount of residual lateral rectus muscle function after recovery. Patients with good residual function have esotropia <20 PD in the primary position with almost full abduction, and those with moderate residual function have esotropia >20 PD with <−2 limitation of abduction. In these patients, ipsilateral medial rectus recession with lateral rectus resection is useful [14]. A posterior fixation suture (Faden) on the contralateral medial rectus (yoke) may be considered for deviation that is much larger in lateral gaze (direction of action of the paralyzed muscle). Patients with larger deviations over 40 PD in primary position may also require recession of the contralateral medial rectus as a staged procedure [28]. Patients with poor or absent residual function have −3 or greater limitation of abduction, some even unable to abduct past the midline. These patients have a negative FGT (discussed in Chap. 6). Resection of an almost fully paralyzed lateral rectus will have little effect, and vertical muscle transposition procedure, with recession of ipsilateral medial rectus, is indicated [29]. Considering the risk of anterior segment ischemia in surgeries involving multiple extraocular muscles, the split tendon transfer procedures are usually preferred than a full tendon transfer procedure [30]. See Text Box 4.1 [31–33]. These procedures are best performed by strabismologists.

Text Box 4.1: Selected Transposition Procedures
Partial tendon transposition (Hummelsheim) [11]: Temporal halves of SR and IR are transposed to LR insertion in LR palsy

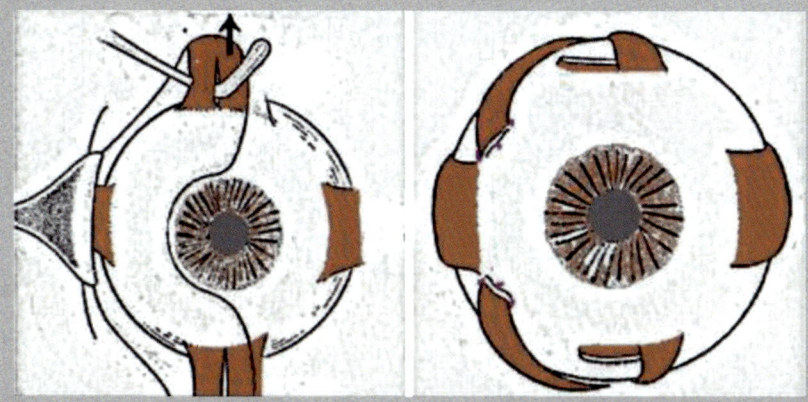

   Rectus muscle union (Jensen) [12]: In LR palsy, the SR, IR, and LR are split along their long axis. The lateral halves of SR and IR are united with superior and inferior halves of LR, respectively.

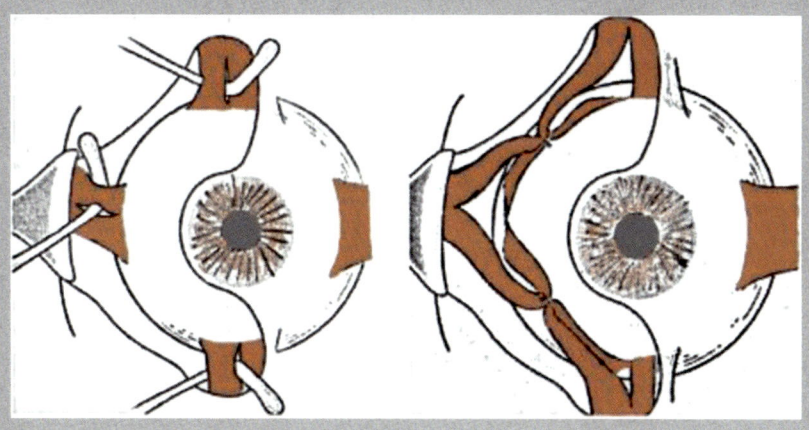

Full tendon transposition for vertical muscle palsy (Knapp) [13]: Both horizontal recti are transposed to the SR in double elevator palsy. The insertions may be placed parallel to the long axis of SR or following the spiral of Tillaux

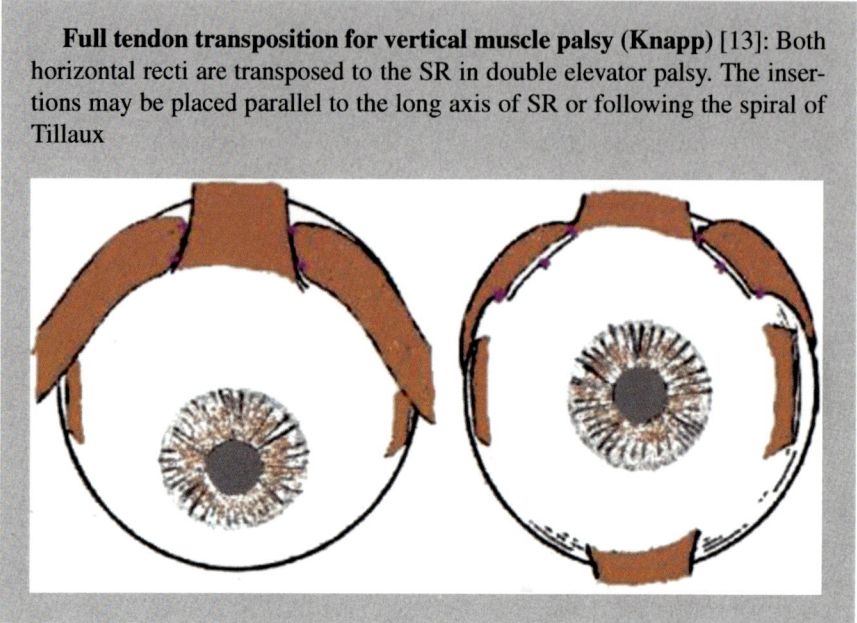

4.6.1.2 Third Nerve Palsy

The surgical treatment of third nerve palsies depends on the number of muscles involved. For single rectus muscle involvement (medial rectus, superior rectus, inferior rectus), the same surgical principle discussed for sixth nerve palsy applies, that is, the amount of residual muscle function guides the decision to perform either recession-resection or muscle transposition. For multiple muscle involvement, surgical plan is decided after assessment of each muscle individually.

For complete third nerve palsies, there are only lateral rectus and superior oblique functioning. The coexisting paralyses of superior rectus, inferior rectus, and medial rectus make tendon transfers from adjacent muscles not feasible. Extreme large lateral rectus recession, sometimes with orbital wall fixation, has been proposed [34]. However, the lateral rectus often reattaches to the globe and creeps forward to result in recurrence of exotropia. Nasal transposition of split lateral rectus can be performed in cases without extensive scarring or lateral rectus contracture from prior muscle surgery [35].

The involvement of levator in third nerve palsy poses another important issue in treatment. The poor or absent levator function often requires frontalis sling procedure to correct the neurogenic ptosis. However, risk of exposure keratitis should be kept in mind in the absence of normal Bell's phenomenon because of paralyzed superior rectus. Some patients develop aberrant regeneration further complicating the situation.

Considering the possibility of troublesome postoperative diplopia and exposure keratitis, careful risk-benefit analysis should be done before initiating treatment [31].

4.6.1.3 Fourth Nerve Palsy

The surgical planning for fourth nerve palsy is complicated due to frequently late presentation with spread of comitance. A general rule is that the surgery is performed on the muscle with greatest overaction in the field of the largest vertical deviation on Hess Chart. Most patients of fourth nerve palsy manifest isolated ipsilateral inferior oblique overaction without obvious superior oblique underaction. Based on this principle, ipsilateral inferior oblique weakening is a frequently performed, effective, and safe initial procedure. Recession of contralateral inferior rectus or recession of ipsilateral superior rectus is performed for larger vertical deviations. When strengthening surgery of superior oblique is indicated, intraoperative exaggerated traction test is performed, and superior oblique tuck is done if tendon laxity is confirmed [36]. These procedures are again best performed by strabismologists.

4.6.2 Restrictive Strabismus

Mechanical restriction results from multiple factors often involving the muscle and its surrounding tissue. Thyroid ophthalmopathy and orbital trauma are the common causes. Surgical management of strabismus in thyroid ophthalmopathy is deferred until the disease is stable. In strabismus associated with trauma, early surgery is advised if significant soft tissue entrapment is visible on imaging.

When definitive surgery is undertaken after control of acute inflammation, preoperative evaluation with forced duction test is important to reveal limitation in duction. The restriction, if clinically significant, is relieved during surgery by release of the scarred or entrapped tissue or by muscle weakening procedure. However, it must be kept in mind that a muscle weakening procedure to correct alignment in the primary position may induce strabismus in the field of action of the weakened muscle which would subsequently require a posterior fixation suture on its yoke muscle [37].

4.6.2.1 Thyroid Eye Disease

Thyroid eye disease (TED) is a self-limited autoimmune inflammatory disorder. Most TED patients have a biphasic course, with an active or progressive phase for up to 18 months, followed by an inactive or stable phase. A characteristic fusiform swelling of the extraocular muscles belly with sparing of tendon on CT scan is often diagnostic. Severe exophthalmos, elevated intraocular pressure, and optic nerve compression may develop and require orbital decompression during the active phase. Strabismus surgery should be considered when the disease has stabilized for 4–6 months and should be delayed until after orbital surgery if necessary.

The surgery is aimed at restoring single binocular vision in primary and downgaze. TED often has both vertical and horizontal deviations (Fig. 4.15). Multiple surgeries are required and adjustable sutures should be used. Traditionally, only recession was recommended for TED; however, resections may also be done for large deviations [38]. Adjustable sutures are often necessary for severe restriction.

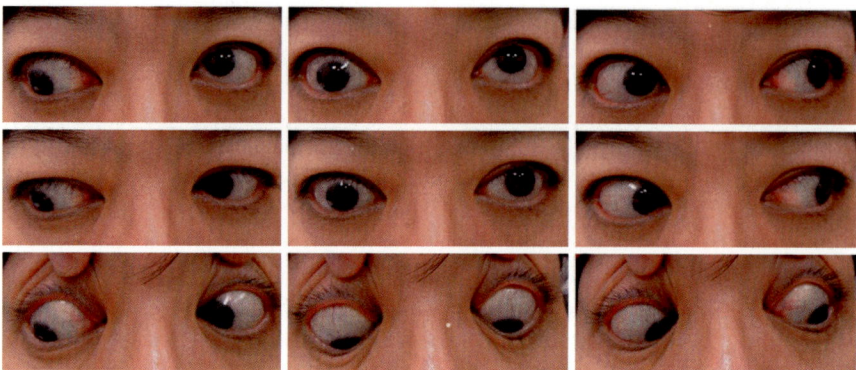

Fig. 4.15 Restrictive strabismus involving right inferior rectus in thyroid eye disease

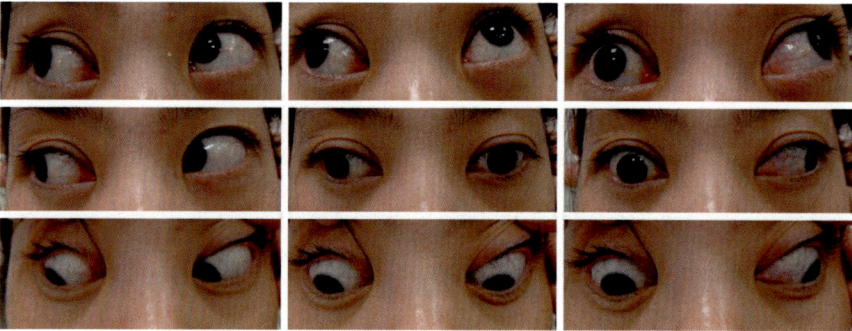

Fig. 4.16 Limitation of elevation and adduction of the right eye after fracture of the orbital floor

The aim should be slight under correction because of the late tendency toward over-correction in TED [39].

4.6.2.2 Orbital Wall Fracture
The strabismus after orbital wall fracture can be caused by muscle injury, muscle entrapment, soft tissue edema, or hemorrhage (Fig. 4.16). Prompt computed tomography (CT) should be obtained to determine extent of orbital fracture and entrapment of ocular tissue. If CT shows clear evidence of extraocular muscle entrapment, early orbital surgery should be considered before permanent tissue changes. If there is no obvious entrapment, the patient may be managed nonsurgically (as discussed earlier). Should troublesome diplopia with no evidence of improvement persist at 6–8 weeks after trauma, strabismus surgery may be considered. However, it must be kept in mind that etiology of strabismus after orbital fracture may be restrictive, paralytic, or combined. The restriction may result from soft tissue fibrosis after original trauma or iatrogenically from orbital wall repair. Recession of the tight muscle and lysis of surrounding fibrotic tissue are usually required. For the paralytic component, the previously described principles for paralytic strabismus should be applied.

4.7 Summary

- It is essential to identify incomitant strabismus as it could be indicative of sinister conditions like intracranial space occupying lesion (SOL).
- Incomitant strabismus can be paralytic or restrictive. Often, both paralytic and restrictive mechanisms coexist in long-standing incomitant strabismus.
- Trauma, microvasculopathies (like diabetes mellitus), thyroid eye disease, viral infections, and SOLs are common causes of acquired incomitant strabismus.
- Larger secondary deviation, diplopia, and anomalous head posture are important clinical features of acquired incomitant strabismus.
- Neuroimaging is indicated in all children presenting with acute-onset strabismus and in adults with pupil involving complete and pupil-sparing *partial* third cranial nerve palsy. Neuroimaging should also be recommended in acquired strabismus in patients below 50 years, non-resolving till 3 months, or aberrant regeneration in non-traumatic palsy.
- Surgical correction is deferred till spontaneous recovery is occurring. Botulinum toxin injection and alternate occlusion may be prescribed during recovery. Surgery is planned to correct the deviation and enhance diplopia-free field in primary and downgazes.
- Choice of surgery is guided by residual motilit in the paralyzed muscle. Muscle transposition surgeries are indicated in completely paralyzed muscles. Adjustable sutures are often used to improve surgical outcomes.
- Early surgery may be needed when restrictive mechanisms are suspected as delay may lead to permanent alterations in extraocular muscle architecture.

4.8 Multiple Choice Questions

1. Which of the following condition is *not* an indication for emergent neuroimaging?
   (a) Pupil involving partial third nerve palsy in adults
   (b) Pupil-sparing complete third nerve palsy in adults
   (c) Acquired sixth nerve palsy in children
   (d) Acquired sixth and seventh nerve palsies in adults

Answer: (b) Pupil-sparing third nerve palsy in adults is usually due to microangiopathy occurring in diabetes mellitus or hypertension. All other conditions commonly occur in central nervous system neoplasms and warrant early imaging.

2. Which of the following is the procedure of choice for right superior oblique palsy with greatest deviation at left upper gaze?
   (a) Right superior oblique tuck
   (b) Right inferior oblique recession
   (c) Left inferior rectus recession
   (d) Right superior rectus recession

Answer: (b) The muscles maximally contracting in left upper gaze are right superior rectus and left inferior oblique (see Chap. 1). Right superior oblique palsy would cause hypertropia with inferior oblique overaction of the right eye. Inferior oblique recession would be indicated for its management.

3. A patient (Fig. 4.17) presented with right sided tilt of the head while walking. He complained of diplopia while going downstairs. All this happened after recovering from the head injury following road traffic accident. On examination there was hypertropia of left eye. The hypertropia worsened in right gaze, with improvement on right tilt. The probable diagnosis is:
   (a) Right SO palsy
   (b) Right SR palsy
   (c) Left SO palsy
   (d) Left SR palsy

Answer: (c) This is a case of acquired Left SO palsy. The test employed to clinch the diagnosis is "Park three-step test".

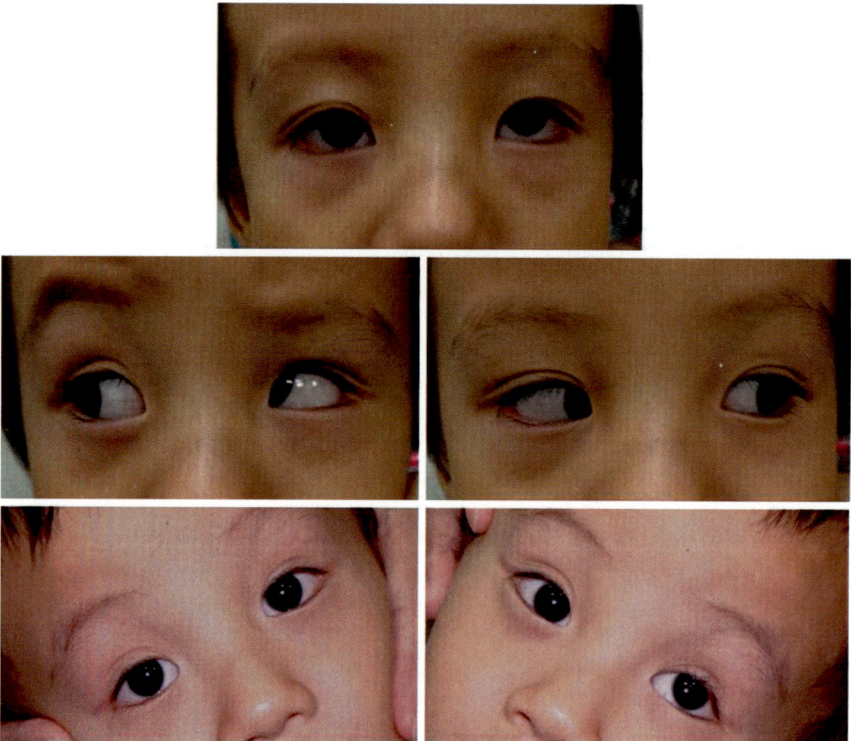

Fig. 4.17 Photography of the patient in Question 3

4. Late clinical findings consistent with an inferior blowout fracture of the orbit include all of the following *except*:
   (a) Proptosis
   (b) Ipsilateral hypotropia on upgaze
   (c) Ipsilateral hypertropia on downgaze
   (d) Positive forced ductions

Answer: (a) In the acute setting, there may be proptosis, but this usually gives way to enophthalmos as swelling subsides.

References

1. Duane A. A new classification of the motor anomalies of the eye based upon physiological principles : together with their symptoms, diagnosis and treatment. New York, NY: J.H. Vail & Co.; 1897. p. 46.
2. Hering E. Die Lehrevombinocularen Sehen. Leipzig: Wilhelm Engelmann; 1869.
3. Tamhankar MA, Volpe NJ. Management of acute cranial nerve 3, 4 and 6 palsies: role of neuroimaging. Curr Opin Ophthalmol. 2015;26(6):464–8.
4. Archer SM, Sondhi N, Helveston EM. Strabismus in infancy. Ophthalmology. 1989;96(1):133–7.
5. Mohney BG, Huffaker RK. Common forms of childhood exotropia. Ophthalmology. 2003;110(11):2093–6.
6. Repka M. Nystagmus surgery. In: Plager D, editor. Strabismus surgery: basic and advanced strategies. New York, NY: Oxford University Press; 2004. p. 162.
7. Parks MM. Isolated cyclovertical muscle palsy. AMA Arch Ophthalmol. 1958;60(6):1027–35.
8. Kushner BJ. Errors in the three-step test in the diagnosis of vertical strabismus. Ophthalmology. 1989;96(1):127–32.
9. Chi SL, Bhatti MT. The diagnostic dilemma of neuro-imaging in acute isolated sixth nerve palsy. Curr Opin Ophthalmol. 2009;20(6):423–9.
10. Miller NR. Solitary oculomotor nerve palsy in childhood. Am J Ophthalmol. 1977;83(1):106–11.
11. Ing EB, Sullivan TJ, Clarke MP, Buncic JR. Oculomotor nerve palsies in children. J Pediatr Ophthalmol Strabismus. 1992;29(6):331–6.
12. Schumacher-Feero LA, Yoo KW, Solari FM, Biglan AW. Third cranial nerve palsy in children. Am J Ophthalmol. 1999;128(2):216–21.
13. Ng YS, Lyons CJ. Oculomotor nerve palsy in childhood. Can J Ophthalmol. 2005;40(5):645–53.
14. Rosenbaum AL, Kushner BJ, Kirschen D. Vertical rectus muscle transposition and botulinum toxin (Oculinum) to medial rectus for abducens palsy. Arch Ophthalmol. 1989;107:820.
15. vonNoorden GK, Murray E, Wong SY. Superior oblique paralysis. A review of 270 cases. Arch Ophthalmol. 1986;104(12):1771–6.
16. Tarczy-Hornoch K, Repka MX. Superior oblique palsy or paresis in pediatric patients. J AAPOS. 2004;8(2):133–40.
17. Parks MM. Management of acquired esotropia. Br J Ophthalmol. 1974;58:240.
18. Robertson DM, Hines JD, Rucker CW. Acquired sixth-nerve paresis in children. Arch Ophthalmol. 1970;83(5):574–9.
19. Aroichane M, Repka MX. Outcome of sixth nerve palsy or paresis in young children. J Pediatr Ophthalmol Strabismus. 1995;32(3):152–6.
20. Lee MS, Galetta SL, Volpe NJ, Liu GT. Sixth nerve palsies in children. Pediatr Neurol. 1999;20(1):49–52.

21. Cox TA, Wurster JB, Godfrey WA. Primary aberrant oculomotor regeneration due to intracranial aneurysm. Arch Neurol. 1979;36(9):570–1.
22. Lyons CJ, Godoy F, AL E. Cranial nerve palsies in childhood. Eye. 2015;29(2):246–51.
23. Volpe NJ, Lee AG. Do patients with neurologically isolated ocular motor cranial nerve palsies require prompt neuroimaging? Journal of neuro-ophthalmology: the official journal of the North American Neuro-Ophthalmology. Society. 2014;34(3):301–5.
24. von Noorden GK, Campos EC. Chapter 20: Paralytic strabismus. In: Binocular vision and ocular motility. 6th ed. St. Louis, MO: Mosby; 2002. p. 414–57.
25. Lee J, Harris S, Cohen J, et al. Results of a prospective randomized trial of botulinum toxin therapy in acute unilateral sixth nerve palsy. J Pediatr Ophthalmol Strabismus. 1994;31:283.
26. Lee JP. Modern management of VI nerve palsy. Aust NZ J Ophthalmol. 1992;20:41.
27. Murray AD. Early botulinum toxin treatment of acute sixth nerve palsy. Eye. 1991;5:45.
28. Rosenbaum AL, Santiago AP. Sixth cranial nerve palsy. In: Clinical strabismus management principles and surgical techniques. Philadelphia, PA: WB Saunders Company; 2001. p. 259–71.
29. Rosenbaum AL. Management of acute and chronic VI nerve palsy. In: Jankovic J, Hallet M, editors. Therapy with botulinum toxin, vol. 387. New York, NY: Marcel Decker; 1995.
30. Couser NL, Lenhart PD, Hutchinson AK. Augmented Hummelsheim procedure to treat complete abducens nerve palsy. J AAPOS. 2012;16(4):331–5.
31. Hummelsheim E. Uber Sehentransplantation an Auge. Ophthal Geselschft. 1907;34:248.
32. Jensen CDF. rectus muscle union: A new operation for paralysis of the rectus muscles. Trans Pac Coast Ophthalmol Soc. 1964;45:359.
33. Knapp P. The surgical treatment of double elevator palsy. Trans Am Ophthalmol Soc. 1969;67:304.
34. Sharma P, Gogoi M, Kedar S, Bhola R. Periosteal fixation in third-nerve palsy. J AAPOS. 2006;10(4):324–7.
35. Shah AS, Prabhu SP, Sadiq MA, Mantagos IS, Hunter DG, Dagi LR. Adjustable nasal transposition of split lateral rectus muscle for third nerve palsy. JAMA Ophthalmol. 2014;132(8):963–9.
36. Rosenbaum AL, Santiago AP. Superior oblique palsy and superior oblique myokymia. In: Clinical strabismus management principles and surgical techniques. Philadelphia, PA: WB Saunders Company; 2001. p. 219–29.
37. Buckley EG, Meekins BB. Faden operation for the management of complicated incomitant vertical strabismus. Am J Ophthalmol. 1988;105(3):304–12.
38. Yoo SH, Pineles SL, Goldberg RA, Velez FG. Rectus muscle resection in Graves' ophthalmopathy. J AAPOS. 2013;17(1):9–15.
39. Harrad R. Management of strabismus in thyroid eye disease. Eye. 2015;29(2):234–7.

Special Variants of Strabismus: Identification and Management Principles

5

Siddharth Agrawal and Rajat M. Srivastava

5.1   Introduction

Occasionally, strabismus not fully conforming to the earlier discussed principles is encountered and requires additional understanding to explain its mechanisms. This chapter will describe several other variants of strabismus which would interest the inquisitive mind of a postgraduate student. A general ophthalmologist should also have their basic knowledge, to identify them and suggest appropriate management.

5.2   A and V Patterns

It has been stressed in earlier chapters that deviation must also be noted in different gazes, for the reason that even comitant horizontal deviations may vary in them. It is not uncommon to find incomitance in vertical gazes in comitant horizontal deviations which presents as A or V pattern.

When eyes appear closer together in upgaze (supra version) compared to downgaze (infra version), the deviation simulates alphabet A, and when the eyes appear closer in downgaze, the deviation simulates alphabet V, hence A and V patterns.

When ET is maximum in upgaze, an A pattern esotropia would result. Similarly, XT maximum in downgaze would cause an A pattern exotropia (Fig. 5.1).

When ET is maximum in downgaze, the esotropia has a V pattern, and when XT is maximum in upgaze, the exotropia has a V pattern (Fig. 5.2).

X, Y and λ patterns may also be observed and are variations of classical A and V patterns [1].

Various theories have been proposed to explain the mechanism of A and V patterns of which the theory of abnormal oblique muscle action is widely accepted. Usually, V

S. Agrawal (✉) · R. M. Srivastava
Department of Ophthalmology, King George's Medical University, Lucknow, India

© Springer Nature Singapore Pte Ltd. 2019
S. Agrawal (ed.), *Strabismus*, https://doi.org/10.1007/978-981-13-1126-0_5

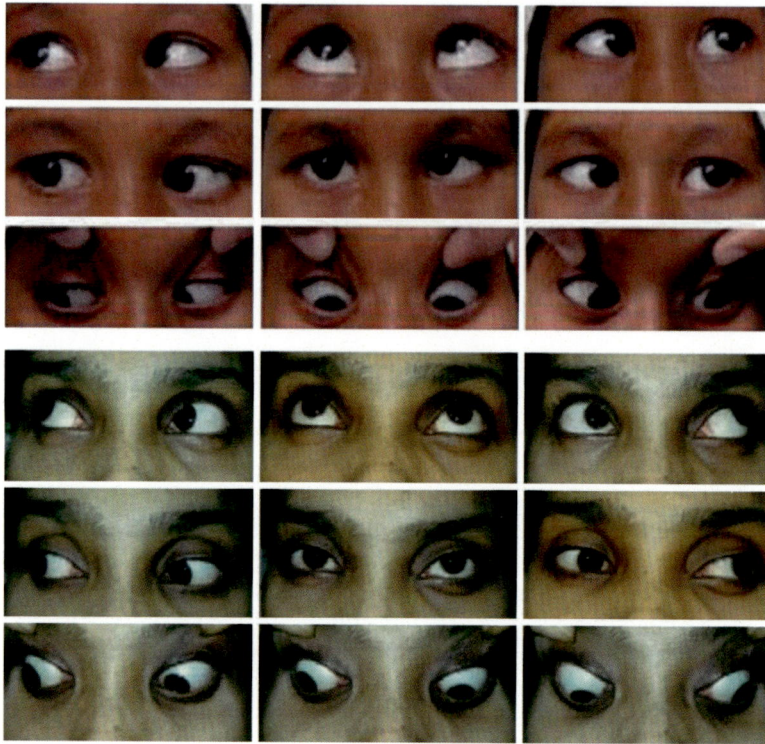

Fig. 5.1 A pattern esotropia (top) and A pattern exotropia (above)

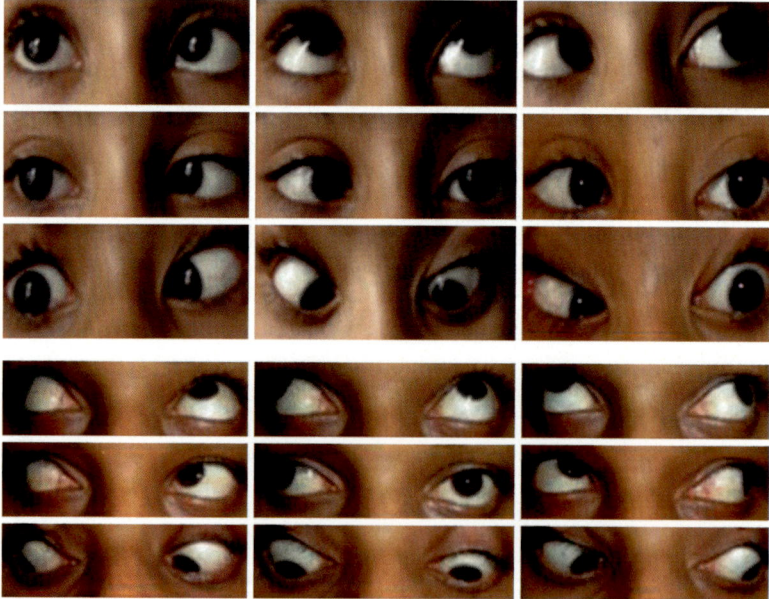

Fig. 5.2 V pattern esotropia (top) and V pattern exotropia (above)

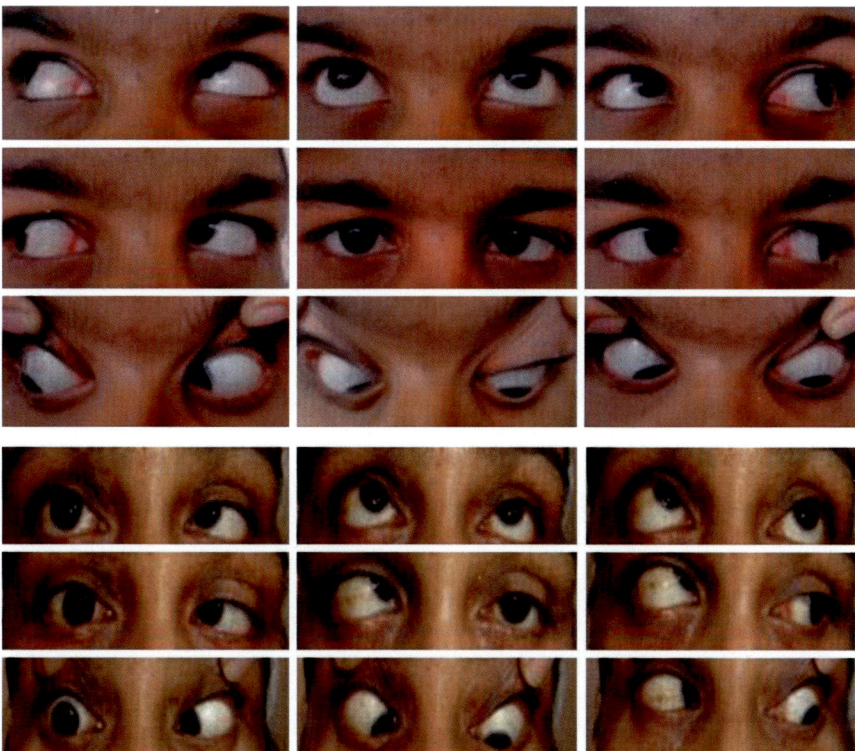

Fig. 5.3 Simple method of grading inferior oblique overaction. The top photographs shows Grade I in RE and Grade II in LE. The bottom photographs shows Grade III in RE

pattern is associated with inferior oblique overaction and A pattern with superior oblique overaction. Grading of inferior oblique overaction is discussed in Chap. 4. A simplified method involves observing whether the inferior oblique overaction (hypertropia) is apparent only when the eye is up and adducted (Grade I) or also when adducted (Grade II) or even in primary gaze (Grade III) as shown in Fig. 5.3. Inferior oblique recession is a commonly performed procedure by strabismus surgeons along with lateral rectus recession for management of V pattern XT. Torsion on fundus photograph may also suggest oblique muscle dysfunction [2] (Fig. 5.4).

A and V patterns can be identified by measuring the horizontal deviation using an accommodative target placed at 33 cm at ~25° above the horizontal plane for upgaze and 35° below the horizontal for downgaze. Slight disparity in horizontal deviation between upgaze and downgaze is physiological. V pattern >15$^\Delta$ and an A pattern >10$^\Delta$ should be considered clinically significant.

This kind of incomitance in comitant deviations poses a challenge, and it should be kept in mind that the downgaze is the most important gaze functionally, after the primary position. Foremost aim of management should be to restore orthotropia and binocularity in these two gazes. It should also be remembered that a V pattern XT and an A pattern ET have the least horizontal deviation in downgaze.

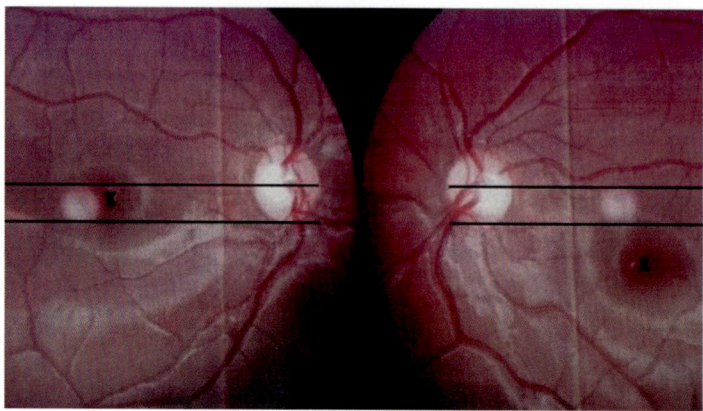

Fig. 5.4 Extorsion of LE in presence of left inferior oblique overaction. Normal location of the fovea is between two imaginary horizontal lines running from the geometric centre of the optic disc and its lower pole. Position of fovea is marked by 'X'. The white shadow in the centre of both pictures is an artefact

With clinically significant pattern deviations, oblique muscle over- or under-actions should be looked for and managed surgically, if present. If this vertical gaze incomitance is not associated dysfunction of oblique muscles, simple modifications like vertical displacement of the horizontal recti or slanting of their new insertion may be done at the time of recession resection surgery. These are discussed in Chap. 8.

> *Clinical Tip: To remember the direction of displacement of horizontal recti for correction of A and V pattern, MR is always shifted to the apex of the 'alphabet' and LR to the base. For example in A pattern, MR is displaced upwards and LR downwards.*

5.3 Dissociated Vertical Deviation (DVD)

DVD is another interesting and challenging condition occasionally encountered in strabismus practice. The condition is called 'dissociated' because unlike the comitant deviations, Herring and Sherrington's laws (Chap. 1) are not followed. To simplify, when the hypertropic eye comes down to take fixation, the already fixing eye does not become hypotropic (but remains straight).

Dissociated vertical deviation (DVD) is usually diagnosed between 2 and 5 years of age and is common in children who have or have been treated for other types of horizontal deviation [3]. Its characteristic is spontaneous up drift of either eye when the patient is inattentive or tired or when fusion is interrupted

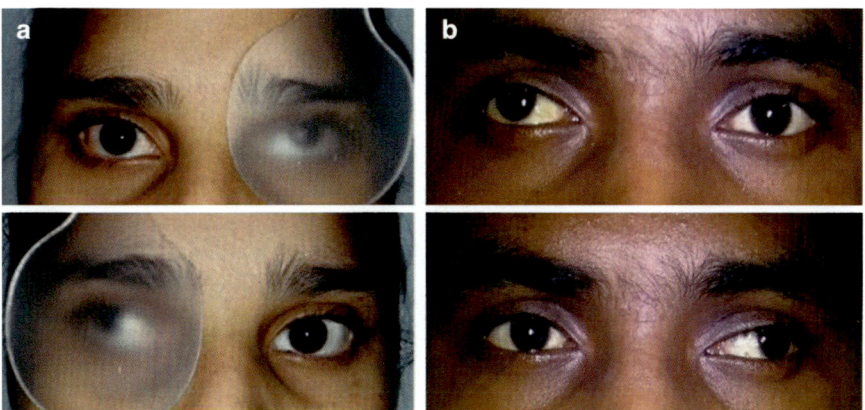

Fig. 5.5 Dissociated vertical deviation. (a) Under cover the left eye predominantly drifts up (DVD) and the right eye drifts both up and out (DVD and DHD). (b) Both eyes have a symmetrical XT, however the right eye also has a DVD

by occlusion of one eye (Fig. 5.5). The condition is usually bilateral and asymmetrical but may occur unilaterally in dense amblyopia and sensory deviations. [4–7]

The symptoms are drifting up of either eye when the patient is tired or 'daydreaming' and asthenopia.

A characteristic Bielschowsky phenomenon has been described for this condition [4] (see the Text Box 5.1). The phenomenon is explained by the tendency of the fixating eye (LE in the example) to drift up when the visual input to it is decreased by neutral density filters. In an effort to maintain fixation against the up drift, innervation to the depressors of fixating eye (LE) increases. The same innervation is received by the (RE) depressors of the eye under cover (Herring's law) which returns to the primary position or even below it. Differential diagnosis of DVD includes inferior oblique overaction.

Text Box 5.1
Bielschowsky phenomenon

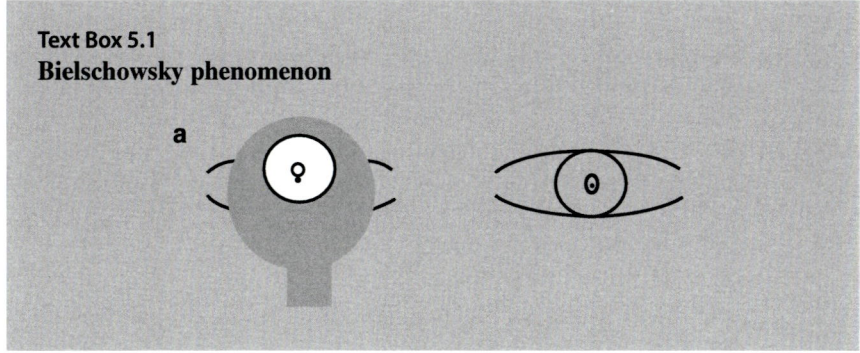

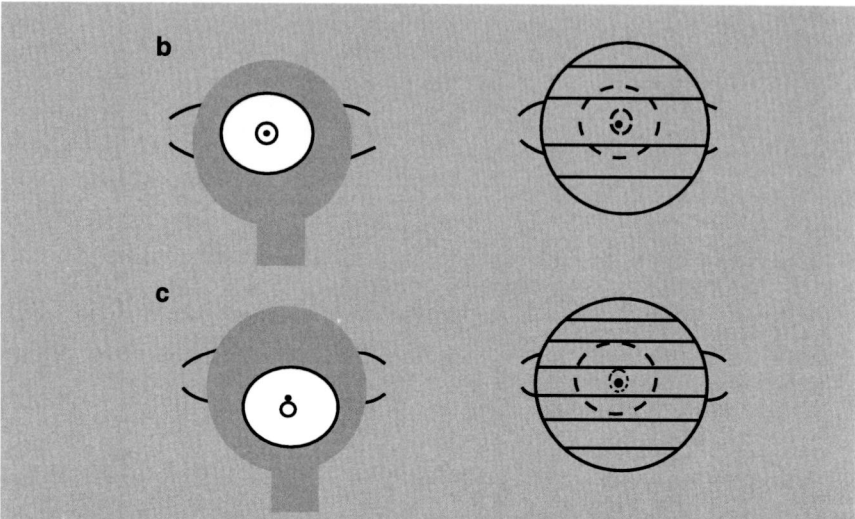

Bielschowsky phenomenon demonstrated in DVD of RE. A translucent occluder is covering the RE while neutral density filters of increasing density are being used to cover the fixing eye (LE): (a) RE up drift under translucent occluder. (b) Neutral density filter placed in front of fixating eye(LE), RE comes down. (c). Filter with greater density causes a down drift of RE.

Differentiating DVD from Inferior Oblique (IO) Overaction

- Upshoot of the eye occurs in maximally in adduction in IO overaction and from any position of horizontal gaze in DVD.
- Superior oblique usually underacts in IO overaction, not so in DVD where it may even overact.
- V pattern is often present in IO overaction.
- Bielschowsky phenomenon and latent nystagmus are often present in DVD.

Another simple test is the placing a red filter in front of either eye, to dissociate them and elicit diplopia. It would be interestingly noted that the patient sees the red image below the fixation light, irrespective of the eye that has the red filter. This is because the eye behind the filter drifts up.

Understanding about this entity is still incomplete, and management options include large recessions of the superior rectus or anterior displacement of the inferior oblique. Recurrences are common.

DVD may be associated with a horizontal component, where the dissociated eye asymmetrically abducts and elevates [8]. This is called dissociated horizontal deviation (DHD) [3, 9].

5.4   Duane Syndrome

Duane syndrome also known as Duane retraction syndrome (DRS) is a form of *congenital incomitant* strabismus characterised by a *small-angle deviation* in primary gaze accompanied by *gross motility limitation* (Fig. 5.6).

DRS is a special form of strabismus described under congenital cranial dysinnervation disorders (CCDD) where the primary findings are nonprogressive and are caused by developmental abnormalities of cranial nerves (or their nuclei) with primary or secondary dysinnervation. It has been found by several researchers, including us, that ipsilateral sixth cranial nerve or its nucleus is dysgenic on Magnetic Resonance Imaging (MRI) in DRS [10, 11].

The symptoms include inability to move an eye in a particular gaze and an anomalous head posture. Often the patient may complain of abnormal narrowing of palpebral aperture or abnormal ocular movement or rarely diplopia. On examination, a gross limitation of abduction with slight limitation of adduction along with globe

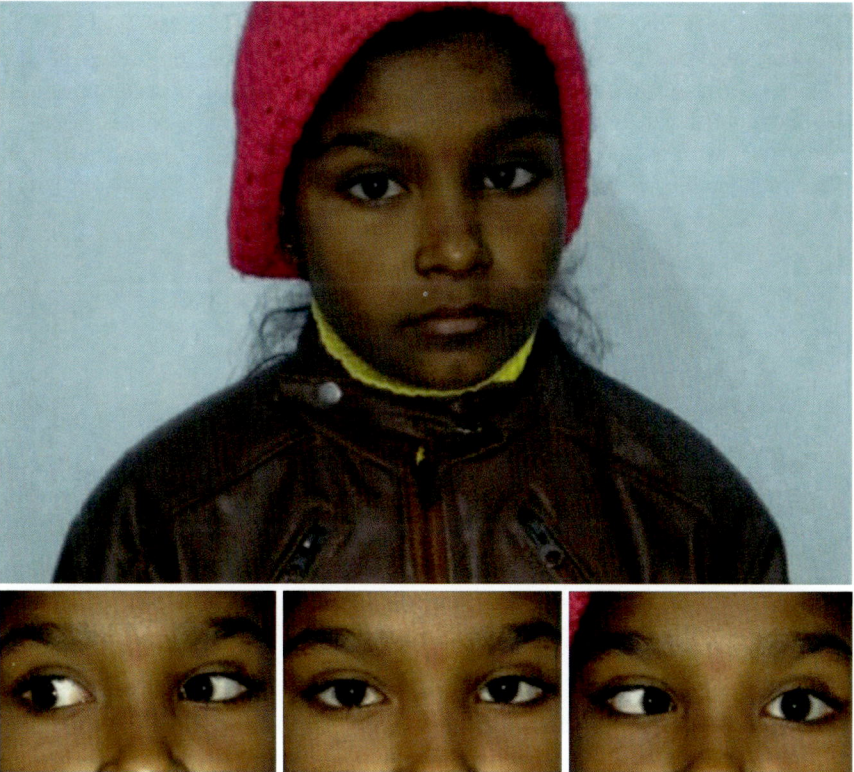

Fig. 5.6 Duane syndrome Type I left eye. Note the anomalous head posture, small-angle deviation in primary position, narrowing of palpebral fissure on adduction and gross limitation of abduction in the left eye

retraction and narrowing of palpebral fissure on adduction is noted. Occasionally up- or downshoot of the eye also is noted on adduction.

Based on motility limitation, three types have been described. Type I in which primarily abduction is limited, in Type II adduction is limited and in Type III both are limited. Type I is commonest and Type II the rarest. ET is commoner in Type I and III and XT in Type II.

This condition must be differentiated from infantile ET and long-standing sixth nerve paresis. Both these conditions have a larger deviation in primary position compared to DRS, but differentiation can often get confusing when patients present as adults. [12]

Surgery should be advised *only* if the deviation in primary position is large (which is rare) or there is significant abnormality of palpebral fissure or a disabling head posture. There is no proven procedure to effectively restore the motility. We have found that surgery is indicated in no more than 10–20% of patients with DRS (unpublished data). Often less experienced surgeons fail to identify this entity and make the patient worse with conventional recession and resection. This should be avoided.

Where indicated, 5 mm recession of the medial rectus of the involved eye is performed in Type I DRS with ET [7]. An asymmetrical recession of the LR of the same side may also be added if globe retraction on adduction is significant [13]. Resection of the lateral rectus should be avoided as it would worsen the retraction. Periosteal fixation of lateral rectus and partial vertical rectus transposition have been shown to be effective in cases of DRS with XT [14]. This however is best left to experts.

5.5   Brown Syndrome

This is a form of restrictive strabismus characterised by absence of elevation in adduction with no limitation of elevation in abduction. The condition may be congenital when it is attributed to anomalies of tendon sheath of superior oblique or acquired after trauma or surgery. The symptoms include limited ocular motility and head posture (Fig. 5.7).

The condition is usually unilateral and forced duction reveals restriction to elevation in adduction of the involved eye. Downshoot on adduction along and a compensatory head posture may also be noted. Hypotropia in primary position may also be noted, specifically after trauma.

Spontaneous remission has been reported in both congenital and acquired cases, hence it is prudent to observe for stability for at least 6 months before surgery is considered [15–17]. Surgery is indicated only in presence of significant deviation in primary position, troublesome diplopia or head posture. Downshoot on adduction, itself is not an indication for surgery. Surgical options include complete tenectomy of the superior oblique or lengthening of the tendon by a silicone expander [18, 19].

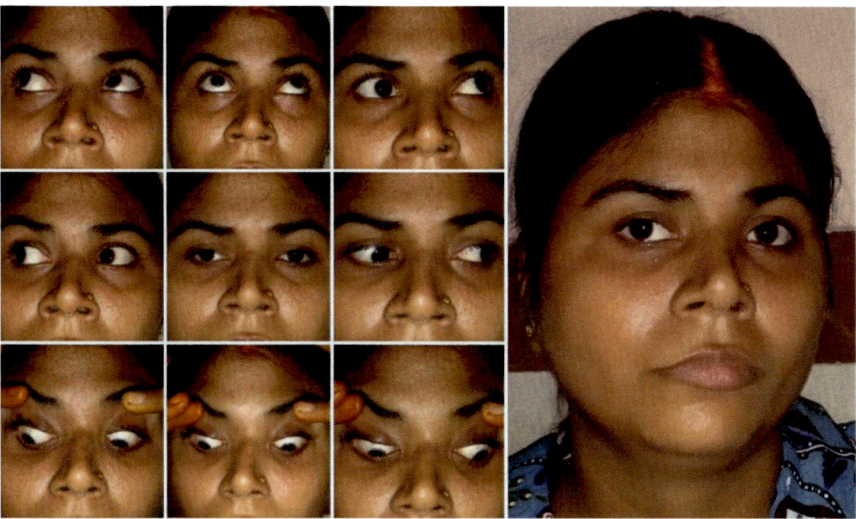

Fig. 5.7 Brown syndrome right eye. Note the anomalous head posture, downshoot on adduction and limitation of elevation in adduction of right eye

5.6   Strabismus Fixus

This is an uncommon type of restrictive strabismus where either one or both the eyes are fixed in extreme adduction (Fig. 5.8). Congenital strabismus fixus patients have been hypothesised to have a fibrotic medial rectus (primary or secondary to lateral rectus palsy). Amyloidosis and high myopia have been implicated in the acquired form [20, 21].

Management involves medial rectus disinsertion or its large recession (on hang back sutures) with resection of the lateral rectus of the involved eye.

5.7   Strabismus Associated with Graves' Disease

Strabismus associated with thyroid ophthalmopathy is usually of restrictive type and may have varied presentations, with restriction of elevation secondary to inferior rectus fibrosis being the commonest (Fig. 4.15). Diplopia, motility limitation and exophthalmos are the usual presenting features (Fig. 5.9). Botulinum toxin can be used as a temporary measure for relief (Chap. 8). Surgery should be performed by experts after stabilisation of the ophthalmopathy. It is discussed in greater detail in Chap. 4. Adjustable sutures are recommended as surgical results are unpredictable.

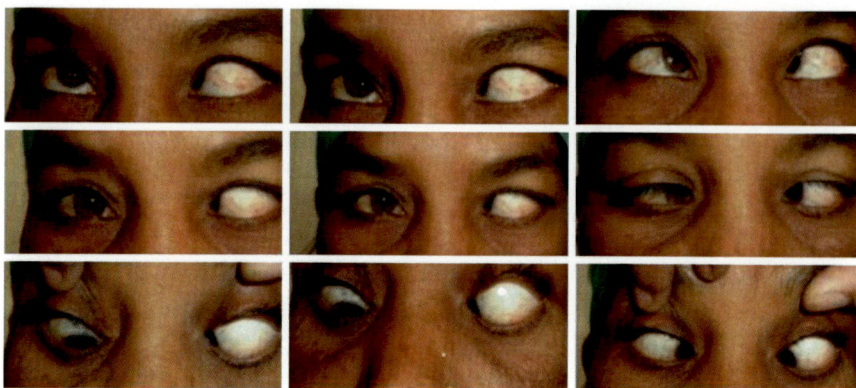

Fig. 5.8 Strabismus fixus LE

Fig. 5.9 Exotropia
associated with Graves'
disease

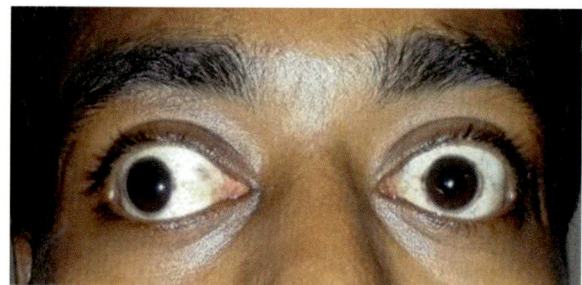

5.8   Cyclic Strabismus

This is a lesser understood type of strabismus which usually follows a 48 h rhythm, i.e. 24 h of manifest heterotropia and 24 h on normalcy (Fig. 5.10). It differs from other types of intermittent deviations as on 'normal' days both the sensory and motor examinations are normal, i.e. the patient has normal binocular vision and there is no latent deviation (phoria). Most common presentation is cyclic esotropia, however occasionally exotropia is also seen. Management consists of observation and surgery if the deviation becomes constant. Surgical alignment according to deviation on 'squinting' days has been suggested for pure cyclic deviations; however, we have no personal experience of performing surgery on these patients [22].

5.9   Nystagmus Associated with Strabismus

5.9.1   Congenital Nystagmus

Congenital nystagmus is broadly classified into manifest and latent (or manifest latent nystagmus (MLN)). Whereas manifest nystagmus is always present, MLN becomes apparent or increases in intensity with occlusion of one eye. Frequently, MLN is

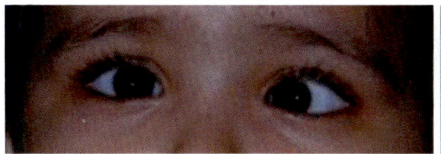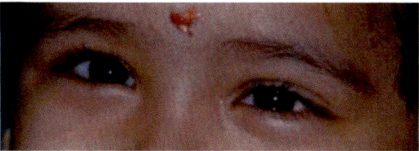

Fig. 5.10 Cyclic strabismus is present on some days only

associated with infantile esotropia. [23, 24] Visual acuity is reduced in almost all patients due to the sensory or neurological cause of nystagmus as well as the nystagmus itself. Usually the acuity is better for near than distance. The table below (Table 5.1) broadly differentiates between manifest and latent types of congenital nystagmus [18, 19].

> *Clinical tip: **Ciancia syndrome** is characterised by uniocular severe visual loss, esotropia, limited abduction and manifest latent nystagmus (MLN). Patient has preferred fixation in adduction and a face turn towards the fixating eye.*

Table 5.1 Differentiating between Manifest and Latent Nystagmus

	Manifest nystagmus	**Latent or manifest latent nystagmus (MLN)**
Common aetiology	Congenital cataract, congenital glaucoma, optic nerve anomaly, oculocutaneous albinism	Unknown, vision loss in 1 eye, strabismus
On occlusion of 1 eye	No change	Increases
Waveform	Biphasic, pendular	Jerking
Slow-phase velocity	Increasing	Decreasing
Strabismus	Occurs rarely	Infantile esotropia frequent
Binocular vs. monocular acuity	Same	Binocular better

5.9.2   Null Zone and Compensatory Head Posture

The position of minimal nystagmus may be straight ahead or in an eccentric direction of gaze. This position is called the null zone or minimal intensity zone [25]. In patients where the null zone is not in primary position, a compensatory head posture is adopted to direct the null zone towards the object of regard.

5.9.3   Nystagmus Blockage or Dampening Syndrome

Frequently, the congenital nystagmus dampens by convergence and the visual acuity improves. In few patients, with early onset variable esotropia, the presentation may vary from ET with no nystagmus when attentive to orthotropia with manifest nystagmus when inattentive. [26] *Nystagmus intensity is believed to be inversely proportional to the angle of deviation.* [27] This is known as nystagmus blockage or dampening syndrome.

5.9.4 Management Principles

Treatment of nystagmus is aimed at improving the visual acuity and correcting the abnormal head posture. There are both non-surgical and surgical options.

1. Refractive correction after cycloplegic refraction is the first step. Myopia over-correction or hypermetropia undercorrection may be attempted to stimulate accommodative convergence.
2. Amblyopia treatment should be done as in children with amblyopia without nystagmus. However, if the nystagmus increases by occlusion of one eye, penalisation may be considered (Chap. 5). It has also been suggested that even if the nystagmus increases, full-time occlusion should be done as the oscillopsia (moving image as perceived by the patient) improves gradually [28].
3. Contact lenses improve nystagmus by improving the acuity as well as with a tactile feedback.
4. Prisms are used to reorient the visual axis so that the eyes remain in the null zone but the head is held straight. Base-out prisms may also be used to stimulate convergence and reduce the intensity of nystagmus.
5. Botulinum toxin type A may be injected into the four horizontal recti (2.5–3 units each) or as a retrobulbar injection (20–25 units) in selected patients to reduce the nystagmus (Chap. 8).
6. Surgical options to correct the horizontal anomalous head posture (in absence of strabismus) are variations of the Kestenbaum-Anderson procedure which recommends a (7 mm) recession of the LR in abducted eye combined with (6 mm) resection of the ipsilateral MR and a (5 mm) recession of the MR of the adducted eye with (8 mm) resection of ipsilateral LR. This is the 5-6-7-8 surgical guideline where each eye receives 13 mm of surgery [26, 29].
7. Large recessions (10 mm for LR and 7.5 mm for MR) of all four horizontal recti have also been suggested to place their insertions behind the functional equator with the aim to dampen the nystagmus and improve visual acuity [26].
8. Bilateral MR recession with or without Faden suture (Chap. 7) is done for nystagmus blockage syndrome.
9. In presence of clinical null zone (or point), surgery is aimed to align the null point to primary position.

5.10 Summary

- Vertical gaze incomitance in horizontal comitant strabismus presents as A and V pattern.
- Inferior oblique overaction is associated with V pattern and superior oblique overaction with A pattern.

- Isolated and independent ocular movements of one or both eyes are seen in dissociated vertical deviations (DVD) and dissociated horizontal deviations (DHD).
- Bielschowsky phenomenon is associated with DVD.
- Duane retraction syndrome (DRS) is a subgroup of congenital cranial dysinnervation disorder (CCDD).
- Elevation restriction in adduction only is a characteristic of Brown syndrome, which is caused by an anomaly of the superior oblique tendon or its pulley.
- Adjustable sutures are commonly used in management of strabismus associated with thyroid ophthalmopathy as the surgical effect is unpredictable.
- Cyclic heterotropia is characterised by alternate periods of strabismus and normalcy.
- Nystagmus blockage syndrome is characterised by esotropia with no nystagmus in an attentive state and orthotropia with nystagmus in an inattentive state.
- Surgical intervention in nystagmus may be done to dampen its intensity, correct the associated strabismus or to bring the null point to primary position.

5.11   Multiple Choice Questions

1. Which of the following is *false* about V pattern exotropia?
   (a) The deviation is maximum in upgaze.
   (b) If associated with Inferior oblique overaction, weakening of inferior oblique is recommended.
   (c) It is commonly associated with superior oblique overaction.
   (d) In normal oblique muscle action, offset or displacement of the horizontal muscle insertion is an option.

Answer (c) V pattern is commonly associated with inferior oblique overaction in presence of which its weakening is done. When oblique muscles are normally acting, displacement or slanting of the horizontal recti insertion is done at the time of surgery. Superior oblique overaction is associated with A pattern.

2. In dissociated vertical deviation, spontaneous up drift of either eye occurs when the patient is inattentive or tired. True about this condition is
   (a) It follows the Herring's law of equal innervation.
   (b) It is usually a unilateral condition seen in infancy.
   (c) Inferior rectus recession is a treatment option.
   (d) Inferior oblique overaction is a differential diagnosis.

Answer (d) DVD does not follow the Herring's law. It is usually a bilateral condition presenting between 2 and 5 years of age. Superior rectus recession and inferior oblique recession are treatment options. Inferior oblique overaction is a differential diagnosis.

3. True about Duane retraction syndrome is
   (a) It has a small-angle deviation in primary position and a gross motility limitation.

(b) It can be differentiated from sixth nerve palsy by difference in motility.

(c) It is currently believed that the extraocular muscle abnormality is responsible for this condition.

(d) Recession-resection surgery in the involved eye works well to correct the deviation and restore motility

Answer (a) It is differentiated from sixth nerve palsy and infantile esotropia by a larger deviation in primary position in these two conditions. Extraocular muscles are normal and the defect lies in the brain stem and origin of sixth nerve. Resection should be avoided in DRS as it worsens the retraction and palpebral fissure abnormality.

4. Regarding management of nystagmus, which of the following statements is *false?*

(a) If nystagmus dampens on convergence overcorrection of myopia or base-out prisms may be tried.

(b) Amblyopia management should not be attempted if occlusion of one eye increases the nystagmus.

(c) Retrobulbar injection of botulinum toxin is an option.

(d) Large recessions of horizontal recti of both eyes may be done.

Answer (b) Amblyopia management should be done. If occlusion increases, the nystagmus and then pharmacological or optical penalisation may be considered.

5. True of Brown's syndrome is

(a) It is a form of paralytic strabismus.

(b) The involved eye does not elevate in abduction.

(c) Forced duction test is positive for superior oblique.

(d) It is usually a congenital condition and requires surgical correction.

Answer (c) Brown's syndrome is a type of restrictive strabismus. The involved eye does not elevate in *adduction* and has a tight superior oblique tendon, demonstrated by a positive FDT. It occurs both as congenital and acquired condition. Surgery is required only in selected cases.

References

1. Hugonnier R, Clayette-Hugonnier S. Strabismus, heterophoria, ocular motor paralysis. Clinical ocular muscle balance. Translated and edited by S Veronneau-Troutman. St Louis, MO: Mosby-Year Book; 1969.
2. Guyton DL. Ocular torsion reveals the mechanisms of cyclovertical strabismus the Weisenfeld lecture. Inves Ophthalmol Vis Scien. 2008;49:847–57.
3. Von Noorden GK, Campos EC. Chapter 18: Cyclovertical deviations. In: Binocular vision and ocular motility. 6th ed. St. Louis, MO: Mosby; 2002. p. 378–84.
4. von Noorden GK. Current concepts of infantile esotropia (Bowman Lecture). Eye. 1988;2:343.

5. Bielschowsky A. Die einseitigen und gegensinnigen ("dissoziierten") Vertikalbewegungen der Augen. Graefes Arch Clin Exp Ophthalmol. 1931;125:493.
6. Romero-Apis D. Comportamiento clinic de los estrabismos secundarios. Anal Soc Mex Oftalmol. 1980;54:153.
7. Sidikaro Y, von Noorden GK. Observations in sensory heterotropia. J Pediatr Ophthalmol Strabismus. 1982;19:12.
8. Brodsky MC. Dissociated horizontal deviation: clinical spectrum, pathogenesis, evolutionary underpinnings, diagnosis, treatment, and potential role in the development of infantile esotropia (an American Ophthalmological Society thesis). Trans Am Ophthalmol Soc. 2007;105:272–93.
9. Wilson ME, McClatchey SK. Dissociated horizontal deviation. J Pediatr Ophthalmol Strabismus. 1991;28(2):90–5.
10. Von Noorden GK, Campos EC. Chapter 21: Special forms of strabimus. In: Binocular vision and ocular motility. 6th ed. St. Louis, MO: Mosby; 2002. p. 458–66.
11. Agrawal S, Singh V, Parihar A, Katiyar V, Srivastava RM, Chahal V. Magnetic resonance imaging (MRI) in Duane retraction syndrome. J Clin Ophthalmol Res. 2016;4:137–41.
12. Agrawal S, Singh V, Agrawal S. Duane syndrome or congenital 6th nerve palsy? Oman J Ophthalmol. 2011;4(2):92–4.
13. Dunlap E. In discussion of Gobin MH: Surgical management of Duane syndrome. Br J Ophthalmol. 1974;58:301.
14. Sharma P, Tomer R, Menon V, Saxena R, Sharma A. Evaluation of periosteal fixation of lateral rectus and partial VRT for cases of exotropic Duane retraction syndrome. Indian J Ophthalmol. 2014;62(2):204–8.
15. Gregersen E, Rindziunski E. Brown's syndrome- a longitudinal long term study of spontaneous course. Acta Ophthalmol Scand. 1993;71:371.
16. Kaban TJ, Smith K, Orton RB. Natural history of presumed congenital Brown's syndrome. Arch Ophthalmol. 1993;111:943.
17. Wang FM, Wertenbaker C, Behrens MM, Jacobs JC. Acquired Brown's syndrome in children with juvenile rheumatoid arthritis. Ophthalmology. 1984;91:23.
18. Sprunger DT, von Noorden GK, Helveston EM. Surgical results in Brown Syndrome. J Pediatr Ophthalmol Strabismus. 1991;28:164.
19. Wright KW. Superior oblique silicone expander for Brown's syndrome and superior oblique overaction. J Pediatr Ophthalmol Strabismus. 1991;28:101.
20. Sharma P, Gupta NK, Arora R, Prakash P. Strabismus fixus convergens secondary to amyloidosis. J Pediatr Ophthalmol Strabismus. 1991;28:236.
21. Bielschowsky A. Das Einwartsschielen der Myopen. Ber Dtsch Ophthalmol Ges. 1922;43:245.
22. Von Noorden GK, Campos EC. Chapter 21:Special forms of strabimus. In: Binocular vision and ocular motility. 6th ed. St. Louis, MO: Mosby; 2002. p. 480–2.
23. von Noorden GK, Munoz M, Wong S. Compensatory mechanisms in congenital nystagmus. Am J Ophthalmol. 1987;104:387.
24. Rosenbaum AL, Santiago AP. Nystagmus: clinical evaluation and surgical management. In: Clinical strabismus management principles and surgical techniques. Philadelphia, PA: WB Saunders Company; 2001. p. 404–18.
25. Abadi RV, Whittle J. The nature of head postures in congenital nystagmus. Arch Ophthalmol. 1991;109:216.
26. Von Noorden GK, Campos EC. Chapter 23: Nystagmus. In: Binocular vision and ocular motility. 6th ed. St. Louis, MO: Mosby; 2002. p. 508–29.
27. Kommerell G. Bezeihungen zwischen strabismus and nystagmus. In: Kommerell G, editor. Disorders of ocular motility: neurophysiological and clinical aspects. Munich: JF Bergmann; 1978. p. 367.
28. Von Noorden GK, Campos EC. Chapter 24: Principles of nonsurgical treatment. In: Binocular vision and ocular motility. 6th ed. St. Louis, MO: Mosby; 2002. p. 537–53.
29. Kestenbaum A. Nouvelle operation du nystagmus. Bull Soc Ophthalmol Fr. 1953;53:599.

Nonsurgical Treatment of Strabismus

6

Siddharth Agrawal, Neha Singh, and Vinita Singh

6.1 Introduction

Previous chapters have highlighted various altered sensory and motor ocular mechanisms associated with strabismus either as cause or effect. The goal of strabismus management is not only to restore motor alignment of the eyes but also to correct any underlying sensory abnormality. While most of the sensory abnormalities are managed conservatively, surgery is often indicated for correcting the static component of the motor misalignment. This chapter will discuss the nonsurgical approach in strabismus management which includes appropriate correction of the refractive error, treatment of associated sensory abnormalities including amblyopia, and treatment of the dynamic component of the deviation.

6.2 Refraction

Cycloplegic refraction should be carried out in all patients having or suspected of having strabismus. Identification and appropriate correction of refractive error is the first essential step before considering any further treatment of strabismus. Prescription of proper glasses provides a sharp retinal image for fusion and creates a balance between accommodation and convergence. It also takes care of the dynamic component of the strabismus and in patients with fully accommodative esotropia may be the only treatment required. Our choice of cycloplegic agent has been discussed in Chap. 1. Here we elaborate the guidelines for prescription of glasses.

Children are most comfortable in their parent's lap and can be made to look straight with the other parent or sibling standing behind the examiner. They may be made to look at distance with screen (even a phone) playing something of their

S. Agrawal (✉) · N. Singh · V. Singh
Department of Ophthalmology, King George's Medical University, Lucknow, India

© Springer Nature Singapore Pte Ltd. 2019
S. Agrawal (ed.), *Strabismus*, https://doi.org/10.1007/978-981-13-1126-0_6

Table 6.1 The American Academy of Ophthalmology Preferred Practice Pattern guidelines for prescribing spectacles in preverbal children

Refractive status	Refractive error (diopter) threshold for correction at different ages		
	≤1 year	1–2 years	2–3 years
Isoametropia (equal or nearly equal refractive error in both eyes)			
Myopia	≥−5.00	≥−4.00	≥−3.00
Hyperopia (no manifest deviation)	≥+6.00	≥+5.00	≥+4.50
Hyperopia with esotropia	≥+2.50	≥+2.00	≥+1.50
Astigmatism	≥3.00	≥2.50	≥2.00
Anisometropia (without deviation)[a]			
Myopia	≥−4.00	≥−3.00	≥−3.00
Hyperopia	≥+2.50	≥+2.00	≥+1.50
Astigmatism	≥2.50	≥2.00	≥2.00

American Academy of Ophthalmology Pediatric Ophthalmology/Strabismus Panel. Preferred Practise Pattern Guidelines. Amblyopia. San Francisco, CA: American Academy of Ophthalmology; 2007. Available from: http://www.aao.org/ppp
Note that in isoametropia, the threshold for correction of hyperopia is higher than myopia in children without strabismus. In presence of esotropia, threshold for hyperopia correction is much lesser.
≤ lesser than or equal to, ≥ more than or equal to
[a]Threshold for anisometropia correction should be lower in presence of deviation

interest. With a little bit of patience, we seldom need to sedate children for retinoscopy and retina examination.

In absence of symptoms or ocular deviation, a hypermetropia of up to + 4 D, myopia up to −3 D, and astigmatism of up to 2 D may be left uncorrected in small children. The American Academy of Ophthalmology Paediatric Eye Evaluations Preferred Practice Pattern summarizes guidelines for prescribing spectacles in children (Table 6.1).

The reader must understand that hypermetropes are overexerting their accommodation to see clear. Accommodation has three components, change in refractive power of crystalline lens, convergence, and miosis, which occur together. The undesired convergence that occurs along with increased accommodative effort to see clear is believed to play a role in certain types of ET [1]. An opposite mechanism would work in myopes who would try to relax their accommodation; however this has a much smaller role in development of XT [2]. Once this is clear, it would also be easy to understand that if abnormally increased convergence occurs with a normal accommodative effort, the eyes would become esotropic on attempts to focus near. This is the etiology of accommodative ET associated with increased AC/A (accommodative convergence/accommodation) ratio.

The unit for AC/A ratio is prism diopter (Δ/diopter (D). Formulae for measuring the AC/A ratio have been listed in Chap. 3.

Clinical Tip: In presence of ET, hyperopia should be maximally corrected to relax any accommodative effort, and in XT, full myopic prescription should be prescribed to induce accommodation.

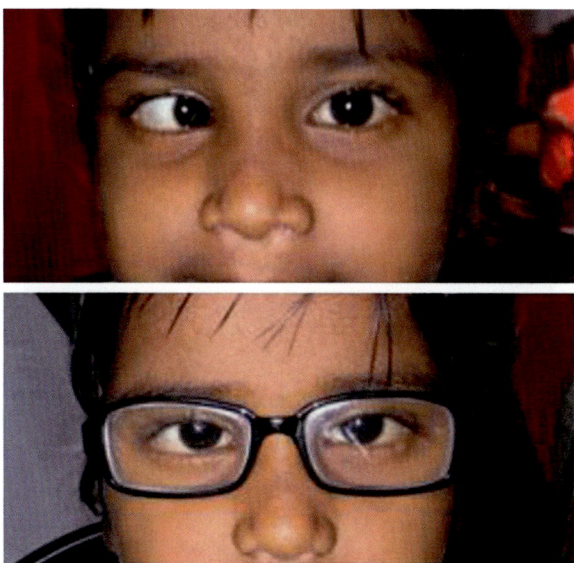

Fig. 6.1 Correction of refractive accommodative esotropia with glasses

In presence of XT, a full or slight overcorrection of myopia and a slight undercorrection of hypermetropia may be desirable. Similarly, in ET, a full correction of hypermetropia should be given [2] (Fig. 6.1). However, an undercorrection of myopia in an attempt to reduce the ET is not desirable [3, 4]. A note should be made of the change in ocular deviation with glasses after allowing suitable time (refractive adaptive time varying from few hours in myopia to few days or weeks in hypermetropia). Where glasses have been deliberately under- or overcorrected and the child complains of asthenopia, a shift toward full correction should be considered. Hypermetropic children may require initial cycloplegia for a few days to adjust to the new glasses [2].

Contact lenses may be prescribed for myopia in older children as placing the refractive correction closer to the nodal point has several advantages in a patient with strabismus [5]. We have reported that strabismus associated with significant anisometropia in young adults may also improve with refractive correction in phakic plane [6, 7].

Bifocals whenever prescribed (in pseudophakes and in ET with high AC/A ratio) should be of pupil bisecting (executive) type only (Fig. 6.2). Progressive lenses should be avoided in children below 12 years of age.

Clinical classification of hypermetropia is depicted in Fig. 6.3, and indications for nonsurgical management of strabismus are listed in Table 6.2.

6.3   Amblyopia

von Noorden defines amblyopia as *"decrease of visual acuity in one eye when caused by abnormal binocular interaction or occurring in one or both eyes as a result of pattern vision deprivation during visual immaturity, for which no cause*

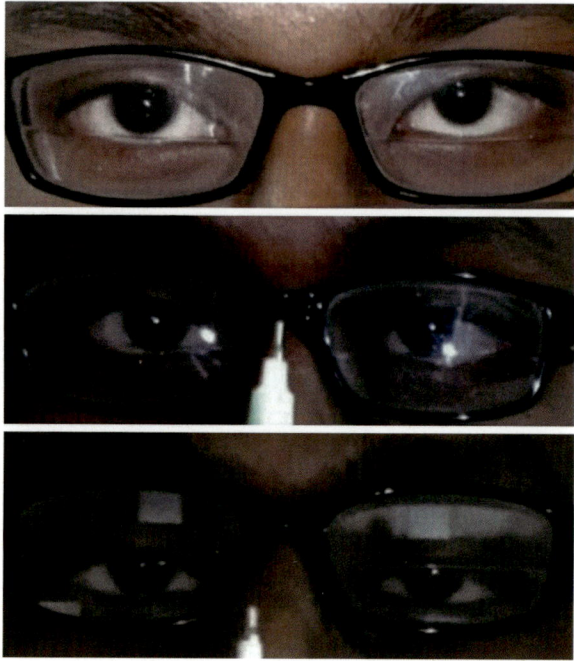

Fig. 6.2 Non refractive accommodative esotropia (with high AC/A ratio). The eyes are ortho-tropic for distance (top). The ET present for near (middle) is corrected when the patient looks through the lower segment of the bifocal lenses (bottom) having just enough addition to convert ET to esophoria

Spherical Error (in Dioptres)	< 2.0	2.25 to 5.0	>5.0
Degree*	Mild	Moderate	High
Clinical Presentation	Latent (detected only after cycloplegia)	Manifest (may be detected without cycloplegia)	
		Facultative (Overcome by accommodation)	Absolute (Always present)
Management	Usually not corrected	Corrected in specific conditions (e.g. symptomatic patient. strabismus, amblyopia)	Corrected

* American Optometric Association. Optometric Clinical Practise Guideline. St.Louis, MO. 2008. Available from https://www.aoa.org/documents/optometrists

Fig. 6.3 Clinical classification of hypermetropia

can be detected during physical examination of the eye(s) and which in appropriate cases is reversible by therapeutic measures." [8]

Simply put (a) an interocular difference of two or more lines or (b) Snellen's single eye best corrected visual acuity lesser than 20/40 or 6/12 (<0.3 logMAR) in the absence of any detectable cause can be termed as amblyopia.

Table 6.2 Indications of nonsurgical treatment of strabismus

1. Refractive errors
2. Sensory abnormalities
(a) Amblyopia
(b) Suppression
(c) Abnormal retinal correspondence
(d) Eccentric fixation
3. Motor abnormalities
(a) Convergence insufficiency
(b) Low fusional amplitude
4. Deviations
(a) Dynamic component, e.g., accommodative ET
(b) Static component, e.g., small-angle deviations, recovering incomitant deviations

Table 6.3 Classification of amblyopia

Based on etiology		
	Abnormal binocular interaction	Vision deprivation
I. Strabismic	Yes	
II. Refractive		
(a) Anisometropic	Yes	Yes
(b) Ametropic	Yes	Yes
III. Stimulus deprivation		
(a) Unilateral	Yes	Yes
(b) Bilateral		Yes
Based on severity	Snellen Acuity (Log MAR)	
I. Mild	>20/40 (<0.3)	
II. Moderate	20/40 to 20/100 (0.3 to 0.7)	
III. Severe	<20/100 (>0.7)	

Amblyopia is caused either by an abnormal binocular interaction or stimulus deprivation during the first 7 years of life (the sensitive period). After this sensitive period, the visual maturation is complete, and the retinocortical pathways become resistant to abnormal visual input [9]. Common causes of amblyopia are strabismus, anisometropia (commoner in anisohypermetropia than anisomyopia), cataract, corneal opacity, or severe ptosis occurring in early childhood. Earlier, longer and denser visual deprivation increases the severity of amblyopia. The classification of amblyopia according to etiology and severity is presented in Table 6.3, and its salient features are listed in Text Box 6.1.

Text Box 6.1: Amblyopia Features
- Caused by abnormal binocular interaction (as in strabismus) or pattern vision deprivation (as in bilateral congenital cataract) or both (as in unilateral congenital cataract).
- Fixation preference for non-amblyopic eye.

- Subnormal near and distance vision.
- Subnormal color vision, contrast, and accommodation.
- Vision improves in mesopic (dim light) conditions.
- Crowding phenomenon (characters appear to run into one another).
- Visual acuity does not improve when tested binocularly (no binocular summation).
- Eccentric fixation.
- Slow and jerky pursuits.
- Larger pupil with increased latency of reaction.

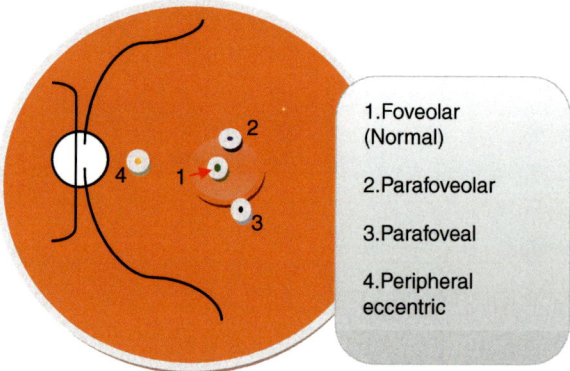

Fig. 6.4 Central (foveolar) and non-foveolar fixation patterns seen in amblyopia [8]

It is the responsibility of each ophthalmologist to diagnose and treat this condition as early as possible. The diagnosis should be one of exclusion when all other organic causes have been ruled out. Once diagnosed, corrected and uncorrected visual acuity for distance and near should be documented. We have seen that if near vision is subnormal and improves with addition of +3.0 D sphere, it implies a weak accommodative effort. This indicates a better prognosis to amblyopia treatment [9]. Effort should also be made to note the fixation with the visuscope attachment of the direct ophthalmoscope (Fig. 6.4).

Anatomical changes in amblyopia have been demonstrated in the lateral geniculate nucleus by von Noorden and in the macular thickness on Optical Coherence Tomography (OCT) by other researchers and us [10, 11]. It would be logical to assume that reversal of these changes would be difficult as the age advances, highlighting the importance of early management.

6.3.1   Principles of Amblyopia Management

After correcting the causative factor, conventional occlusion of the non-amblyopic eye remains the gold standard treatment. Few points to be remembered while treating amblyopia are:

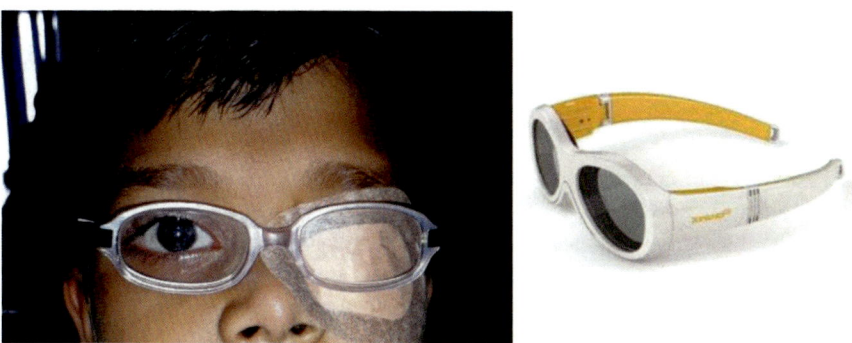

Fig. 6.5 Amblyopia treatment. While occlusion of the non-amblyopic eye remains the gold standard, newer options like digital amblyopia goggles are emerging

1. Occlusion or atropine penalization may not be started immediately with the prescription of glasses for the first time. It would come as a shock to the child and the parents who would tend to become non-compliant. Moreover, it has been shown that large percentage of children with mild to moderate anisometropic amblyopia improve two or more lines of vision within 15 weeks of wearing glasses alone [12]. Subsequently, occlusion or penalization should be started in children who do not show full improvement.

2. Occlusion should be done directly with a patch so that the child does not peek through the side of glasses (Fig. 6.5).

3. Initially full-time occlusion was prescribed in all children. This had poor compliance, dissatisfied parents, and also the risk of occlusion amblyopia of the sound eye.

    The recommendations of Pediatric Eye Disease Investigator Group (PEDIG) are that moderate amblyopia (20/40–20/100) responds well to 2 h/day patching and severe amblyopia (20/100–20/400) responds to 6 h/day patching of the sound eye [13, 14]. It should be kept in mind that these regimens are effective when initiated below 5 years of age, with proper compliance and the children actively using the amblyopic eye during the period of occlusion [15–17].

4. Suitable correction should be worn over the amblyopic eye, and the child should be encouraged to perform near work like coloring or playing video games when the better eye is occluded.

5. Follow-ups should occur every 4 weeks to monitor change in visual acuity and fixation preference. No improvement should raise the suspicion of improper technique. We believe that pleoptics or office exercises to stimulate the amblyopic macula only serve to reduce missed appointments by patients.

6. Weekend atropine penalization of the sound eye was initially suggested as an option in children non-compliant to occlusion or in maintenance phase but is now recommended as an alternative to occlusion in primary amblyopia management [18–21]. *Penalization* of the sound eye combined with overcorrection of the amblyopic eye by +1.0 to +3.0 D sphere forces the child to use the amblyopic eye for near work [4].

7. Miotics may be used as an alternative to hypermetropic glasses in the amblyopic eye, to facilitate accommodation without effort in children non-compliant to glasses. The same principle is followed in prescription of miotics as an alternative to bifocals in accommodative ET.
8. Although best response is seen in children below 6 years of age, a sincere attempt to improve vision in the amblyopic eye must be made in older children and even adults. We have seen vision improve in adults over 20 years of age.
9. As the vision starts to improve, attempts must be made to assess and improve the binocular functions. Ocular alignment may be considered as the improvement begins, as alignment itself enhances the response to treatment, provided amblyopia therapy is continued after surgery [22]. If parents are non-compliant, it may be prudent to wait for surgery till complete recovery of vision in the amblyopic eye.
10. Several newer options like digital amblyopia goggles are available, but we have a limited experience with these (Fig. 6.5). A randomized trial addressing this issue is lacking. Considering the initial cost and recurring cost of maintenance in an active child, they are unlikely to become very popular. Binocular visual stimulation through the use of dichoptic glasses while playing video games is the newest treatment regimen which appears promising [23].
11. Drugs like levodopa should not be used [24, 25]. Citicoline appears to be promising and may be given in selected patients [26].
12. After complete resolution gradual tapering of the treatment should be continued till 8–10 years of age. Recurrence is common if the treatment is stopped abruptly [27].

In presence of nystagmus which increases on occlusion, overcorrecting the hyperopia or using lightly frosted glasses (achievable by applying neutral colored nail paint on glass) in the sound eye to reduce its vision to one line below the amblyopic eye may be advisable. We have found this to serve the purpose of occlusion without increasing the nystagmus. However, some researchers advocate full-time occlusion and believe that the oscillopsia improves gradually [4]. Penalization is also effective.

> *Clinical Tip: In presence of strabismic amblyopia, amblyopia therapy should be rigorously initiated prior to surgical alignment and be continued thereafter* [22].

6.4 Orthoptics

Once amblyopia has been overcome, subsequent efforts are directed at strengthening of binocular fusion as achieving normal binocular single vision (BSV) is the ultimate aim of strabismus management. Binocular vision better than uniocular

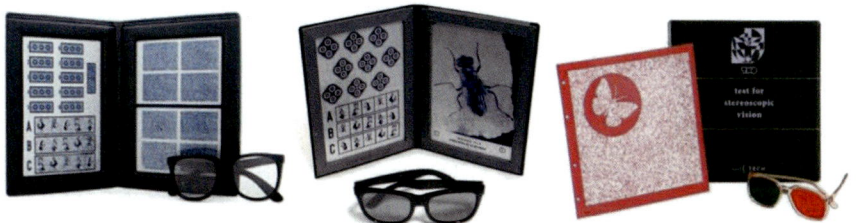

Fig. 6.6 Quantification of stereopsis. Left to Right. Random Dot, Titmus fly, and TNO test. These tests are performed after dissociating the two eyes with polaroid or red green glasses

Table 6.4 Grades of Binocular Single Vision (BSV)

Simultaneous Macular Perception (SMP): ability to perceive separate stimuli at the same time			
Fusion: unification of visual impulses from the corresponding retinal images into a single visual percept. To simplify, the ability to fuse (as 1) slightly dissimilar images falling on *corresponding retinal points* of two eyes			
Average fusional amplitudes (vergence in prism diopters)			
	Convergence	Divergence	Vertical
Distance	14	6	2.5
Near	38	16	2.6
Stereopsis: is binocular appreciation of an object in *depth* due to fusion of images that stimulate *horizontally disparate retinal points*			
Normal range of stereopsis			
Distance	200–450 s of arc		
Near	20–40 s of arc		

vision (binocular summation), ability to appreciate physiological diplopia, and correct response on Worth Four Dot Test (WFDT) confirm the presence of binocular single vision (BSV). These tests can be performed in the office of each ophthalmologist without the need of any special equipment.

Grading binocular vision requires a synoptophore, and quantification of stereopsis is done by tests like Titmus Stereo, TNO, or Random Dot (Fig. 6.6 and Table 6.4) [28]. Assessment of binocular functions has been dealt in Chap. 2.

Satisfactory motor alignment and good vision in each eye are primary requirements for BSV. Motor alignment enables the images to fall within the Panum's area which itself provides a stimulus for binocular fusion and stereopsis. This may be further reinforced by orthoptic exercises.

Literal meaning of the word "orthoptics" is "straight sight." Truly speaking, entire strabismus examination and all nonsurgical treatment including amblyopia management is orthoptics, which is carried out by the treating physician or under his direct supervision.

The role of the orthoptist and the synoptophore is limited to the following in current scenario:

1. Confirming the deviation preoperatively

This is more relevant in vertical and torsional deviations measurements of which are better performed on the synoptophore.

2. Convergence and fusion exercises

An individual with normal convergence should be able to converge his eyes and see an object like pencil tip clearly at about 10 cm for 30 s. Those unable to do this may be symptomatic because of convergence insufficiency.

Convergence exercises prescribed in presence of convergence insufficiency are effective. The patient is taught to converge on an object like a pen at the closest distance that he can see clearly. At the same time, he is made aware of physiological diplopia for distance objects. The patient is then asked to remove the near object, while continuing to voluntarily converge and have diplopia for distance. In subsequent attempts the distance at which the pen is initially held is gradually reduced. This exercise should be performed for not more than 5 min and never when the patient is tired or sleepy.

Fusion exercises are performed on the synoptophore or with prisms by an orthoptist. They are useful to increase the fusional range in patients with subnormal fusional amplitude.

3. Pleoptics

Several exercises and equipment have been described to actively stimulate the macula, like the CAM stimulator and the Haidinger's brushes. They have a limited utility except to encourage the patients to regularly attend the follow-up visits.

6.5   Prisms

Prisms have a therapeutic utility in facilitation of binocular vision in small-angle deviations, especially in residual or consecutive deviations postsurgery. Prisms can be incorporated in lenses with prescription or may be stuck on their back surface (Fresnel prisms). While prescribing, the base of the prism should point away from the deviation, for example, base in prisms would be prescribed in XT. Also, the total amount of prisms to be prescribed in prism diopters (Δ) should be divided between the two eyes. Prescription of prisms is best left to the specialist.

6.6   Chemodenervation

Chemodenervation with botulinum toxin has been discussed in detail in Chap. 9.

6.7   Summary

NON SURGICAL MANAGEMENT OF STRABISMUS

OPTICAL

PHARMACOLOGIC

ORTHOPTICS (including Amblyopia Management)

1. Spectacles

Esodeviations

- Hypermetropes: full correction
- Myopes: full correction
- High AC/A ratio: bifocals

Exodeviations

- Myopes: full /overcorrection
- Hypermetropes: undercorrection

2. Prisms
- Glass: upto 8Δ
- Fresnel: upto 30 Δ

1. Cycloplegics

- Facilitate acceptance of hypermetropic correction in children
- Accommodative ET (rarely used)

2. Miotics

- Esodeviations with high AC/A ratio
- Amblyopia therapy

3. Chemodenervation
- Botulinum toxin

1. Amblyopia management

- Occlusion
- Penalisation
- Binocular visual stimulation
- Drugs (e.g.citicholine)

2. Convergence and fusion exercises

3. Pleoptics

4. Prisms and occlusion in incomitant deviations

6.8   Multiple Choice Questions

1. Amblyopia is decreased visual acuity in the absence of any obvious cause. True statement with regard to it is:
   (a) It is almost always unilateral.
   (b) Anisometropia would cause it to be denser compared to total congenital cataract.
   (c) Strabismus would cause it to be denser compared to total congenital cataract.
   (d) Unilateral congenital cataract would cause it to be denser compared to bilateral.

Answer (d) Amblyopia is frequently bilateral. Congenital cataract causes form vision deprivation unlike strabismus and anisometropia which cause abnormal binocular interaction. Amblyopia due to vision deprivation is denser. Unilateral congenital cataract causes both form vision deprivation and abnormal binocular interaction; as a result it causes one of the densest amblyopia.

2. Amblyopia is reversible if treated in time and appropriately. A good prognostic sign for amblyopia is:
   (a) Established eccentric fixation
   (b) Visual deprivation occurring at an early age
   (c) Near vision improves with +3.0 D sphere
   (d) Detection during college entrance medical examination

Answer (c) Established eccentric fixation, early visual deprivation, and late detection are all poor prognostic. Improved near vision is suggestive of impaired accommodation and carries good prognosis [9].

3. Orthoptic exercises should be best considered in management of:
   (a) Convergence insufficiency
   (b) Infantile esotropia
   (c) Dissociated vertical deviation
   (d) Sixth nerve paralysis

Answer (a) Orthoptic exercises are treatment of choice for symptomatic convergence insufficiency. They are not indicated in other three conditions.

4. Accommodative esotropia with high AC/A ratio is best managed by:
   (a) Progressive glasses
   (b) Executive type bifocals
   (c) Full hypermetropic correction
   (d) Surgery

Answer (b) In patients of accommodative esotropia with convergence excess (high AC/A), a full correction for distance will leave residual esotropia for near which should be corrected with near addition. Executive type bifocals (large lower segment bisecting the pupil) are preferred in children.

5. A 4-year-old child presents with left esotropia and amblyopia. What is the correct sequence of management?
   (a) Cycloplegic refraction → amblyopia therapy → Squint surgery
   (b) Cycloplegic refraction → squint surgery → amblyopia therapy
   (c) Cycloplegic refraction → amblyopia therapy only
   (d) None of the above

Answer (a) Cycloplegic refraction is always the initial step in management of comitant strabismus. Ocular alignment should be considered only after completion of amblyopia management.

6. Correct statement regarding prescription of glasses in intermittent exotropia:
   (a) Hypermetropia may be overcorrected to control deviation.
   (b) Myopia should always be fully corrected.
   (c) Undercorrection of hypermetropia and overcorrection of myopia may help to control deviation.
   (d) Both (b) and (c)

Answer (d) Myopia should always be fully corrected in exotropia to help in fusion. A slight overcorrection of myopia and a slight undercorrection of hypermetropia may be desirable to increase accommodative effort which would subsequently increase convergence and help in controlling the deviation.

References

1. von Noorden GK, Campos EC. Chapter 16: Esodeviations. In: Binocular vision and ocular motility. 6th ed. St. Louis, MO: Mosby; 2002. p. 311–49.
2. von Noorden GK, Campos EC. Chapter 17: Exodeviations. In: Binocular vision and ocular motility. 6th ed. St. Louis, MO: Mosby; 2002. p. 356–76.
3. American Academy of Ophthalmology. Chapter 9: Exodeviations. In: Basic and clinical science course. Pediatric ophthalmology and strabismus 2015-16. San Francisco, CA: American Academy of Ophthalmology; 2015. p. 99–107.
4. Von Noorden GK, Campos EC. Chapter 24: Principles of nonsurgical treatment. In: Binocular vision and ocular motility. 6th ed. St. Louis, MO: Mosby; 2002. p. 537–53.
5. Herman JS, Johnson R. The accommodation requirement in myopia. A comparison of contact lens and spectacles. Arch Ophthalmol. 1966;76:47–51.
6. Agrawal S, Singh V, Yadav A, Katiyar V. Orthoptic relevance of refractive correction in the phakic plane in unilateral high refractive errors in adults. Oman J Ophthalmol. 2016;9:196–8.
7. Agrawal S, Singh V. Correction of exotropia by implantable collamer lens (ICL). Indian J Ophthalmol. 2013;61:685.

8. von Noorden GK, Campos EC. Chapter 14: Amblyopia. In: Binocular vision and ocular motility. 6th ed. St. Louis, MO: Mosby; 2002. p. 246–86.
9. Singh V, Agrawal S. Visual functions in amblyopia as determinants of response to treatment. J Pediatr Ophthalmol Strabismus. 2013;50(6):348–54.
10. Yen MY, Cheng CY, Wang AG. Retinal nerve fiber layer thickness in unilateral amblyopia. Invest Ophthalmol Vis Sci. 2004;45(7):2224–30.
11. Agrawal S, Singh V, Singhal V. Cross sectional study of macular thickness variations in unilateral amblyopia. J Clin Ophthalmol Res. 2014;2(1):15–7.
12. Cotter SA, Edwards AR, Wallace DK, et al. Pediatric Eye Disease Investigator Group. Treatment of anisometropic amblyopia in children with refractive correction. Ophthalmology. 2006;113(6):895–903.
13. Repka MX, Beck RW, Holmes JM, et al. Pediatric Eye Disease Investigator Group. A randomized trial of patching regimens for treatment of moderate amblyopia in children. Arch Ophthalmol. 2003;121(5):603–11.
14. Holmes JM, Kraker RT, Beck RW, et al. Pediatric Eye Disease Investigator Group. A randomized trial of prescribed patching regimens for treatment of severe amblyopia in children. Ophthalmology. 2003;110(11):2075–87.
15. Scheiman MM, Hertle RW, Beck RW, et al. Pediatric Eye Disease Investigator Group. Randomized trial of treatment of amblyopia in children aged 7 to 17 years. Arch Ophthalmol. 2005;123(4):437–47.
16. Repka MX, Kraker RT, Beck RW, et al. Pediatric Eye Disease Investigator Group. A randomized trial of atropine vs patching for treatment of moderate amblyopia: follow-up at age 10 years. Arch Ophthalmol. 2008;126(8):1039–44.
17. Holmes JM, Lazar EL, Melia BM, et al. Pediatric Eye Disease Investigator Group. Effect of age on response to amblyopia treatment in children. Arch Ophthalmol. 2011;129(11):1451–7.
18. Pediatric Eye Disease Investigator Group. A randomized trial of atropine vs. patching for treatment of moderate amblyopia in children. Arch Ophthalmol. 2002;120(3):268–78.
19. Repka MX, Wallace DK, Beck RW, et al. Pediatric Eye Disease Investigator Group. Two-year follow-up of a 6-month randomized trial of atropine vs patching for treatment of moderate amblyopia in children. Arch Ophthalmol. 2005;123(2):149–57.
20. Repka MX, Cotter SA, Beck RW, et al. Pediatric Eye Disease Investigator Group. A randomized trial of atropine regimens for treatment of moderate amblyopia in children. Ophthalmology. 2004;111(11):2076–85.
21. Repka MX, Kraker RT, Beck RW, et al. Pediatric Eye Disease Investigator Group. Treatment of severe amblyopia with weekend atropine: results from 2 randomized clinical trials. J AAPOS. 2009;13(3):258–63.
22. Lam GC, Guyton DL. Timing of amblyopia therapy relative to strabismus surgery. Ophthalmology. 1993;100(12):1751–6.
23. Hess RF, Mansouri B, Thompson B. A new binocular approach to the treatment of amblyopia in adults well beyond the critical period of visual development. Restor Neurol Neurosci. 2010;28:793–802.
24. Repka MX, Kraker RT, Dean TW, et al. Pediatric Eye Disease Investigator Group. A randomized trial of levodopa as treatment for residual amblyopia in older children. Ophthalmology. 2015;122(5):874–81.
25. Hoyt C. What is next in amblyopia treatment? Ophthalmology. 2015 May;122(5):871–3.
26. Pawar PV, Mumbare SS, Patil MS, et al. Effectiveness of the addition of citicoline to patching in the treatment of amblyopia around visual maturity: a randomised controlled trial. Indian J Ohthalmol. 2014;62:124–9.
27. Holmes JM, Beck RW, Kraker RT, et al. Pediatric Eye Disease Investigator Group. Risk of amblyopia recurrence after cessation of treatment. J AAPOS. 2004;8(5):420–8.
28. von Noorden GK, Campos EC. Chapter 15: Examination of patient V. Depth perception. In: Binocular vision and ocular motility. 6th ed. St. Louis, MO: Mosby; 2002. p. 298–304.

Planning Strabismus Surgery

Rolli Khurana, Neha Singh, Rajat M. Srivastava, and Siddharth Agrawal

7.1   Introduction

After a conclusive diagnosis has been made, meticulous surgical planning and its execution form the final steps in successful management of strabismus. This chapter will highlight the points to be considered while planning strabismus surgery.

While achieving a near perfect alignment of visual axes is the aim, ocular alignment in at least the primary and downgaze is most desirous (Table 7.1). This may be achieved by either "correcting the defect" or by "matching the defect" of the sound eye to the squinting eye. At the same time, all considerations must also be made to ensure sensory recovery as achieving good binocular functions is the ultimate goal of any strabismus surgery. Binocular function recovery depends on multiple factors like vision, age of onset, duration and stability of deviation along with preoperative binocular functions (Table 7.2). An adult with early-onset, long-standing, constant (no intermittency or variability) deviation with poor vision in deviating eye and poor binocular functions can be expected to have an unfavourable prognosis in terms of sensory recovery [1].

The surgeon should also spend time to understand the expectations of the patient and see if they match with the expected surgical outcome. This would avoid disappointment and hours of postoperative counselling.

R. Khurana
Dr Shroff's Charity Eye Hospital, Delhi, India

N. Singh · R. M. Srivastava (✉) · S. Agrawal
Department of Ophthalmology, King George's Medical University, Lucknow, India

© Springer Nature Singapore Pte Ltd. 2019
S. Agrawal (ed.), *Strabismus*, https://doi.org/10.1007/978-981-13-1126-0_7

Table 7.1 Management goals of strabismus treatment

Sensory
1. Restoration of normalcy of visual acuity
2. Achieve normal stereopsis and fusional range in all gazes and if that is not possible then in functional positions, i.e. primary and downgaze
Motor
1. In ET—Orthotropia (ideal) but if unachievable then microtropia or deviation ± 10 PD of orthotropia is also satisfactory
2. In XT—Small consecutive ET with diplopia (except in small children)
3. In sensory deviations—Small angle ET

Table 7.2 Factors affecting binocular recovery (binocular potential) after strabismus surgery [1]

1. Age of onset
2. Duration
3. Intermittency
4. Variability
5. Vision
6. Preoperative binocularity

7.2   Anatomical Considerations

A clear understanding of the surgically relevant anatomy is the prime prerequisite for satisfactory surgical outcomes (Figs. 7.1 and 7.2). A thorough familiarity with the orientation of the extraocular muscles (EOM) in the orbit and relative to the eyeball is a must.

7.2.1   The Recti

The recti, after traversing their course along the orbital walls, pierce the Tenon's capsule 8–10 mm from their insertions into the sclera. It is in this episcleral space where the muscles are manipulated at their insertions.

7.2.1.1 Medial Rectus Muscle

Medial rectus (MR) has a relatively straight course, a short arc of contact and minimal surrounding attachments, making it most prone to retract posteriorly if the surgeon loses control of the muscle after its disinsertion from the sclera [2, 3]. Muscle may also slip intraoperatively or postoperatively if the suture placement is too superficial and does not incorporate the entire tendon thickness.

Oculocardiac reflex (detailed in next chapter) is commonest with MR muscle. The anaesthetist should be informed while manipulating this muscle.

7.2.1.2 Lateral Rectus Muscle

Due to better exposure of the temporal side of the eyeball, surgical dissection of lateral rectus (LR) is easier compared to MR. Being a long and thin muscle, care

Fig. 7.1 Axial view depicting anatomical relation of the right eyeball with respect to orbit and extraocular muscle insertions

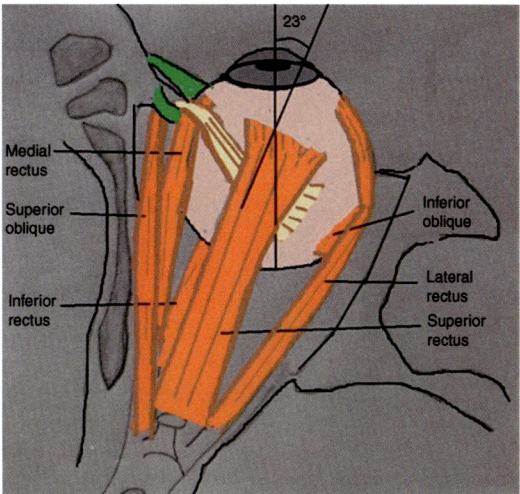

Fig. 7.2 Sagittal section of the globe showing attachments of vertical recti with lids

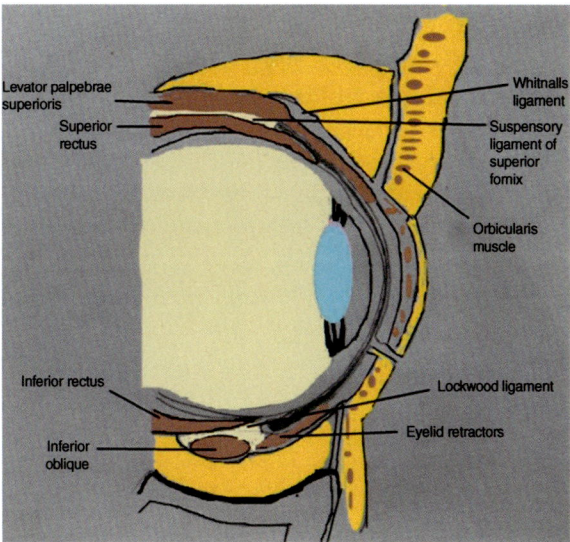

should be taken while hooking its fibres so as to not split them. Moreover, the inferior oblique may be inadvertently hooked or damaged due to the presence of loose fascial attachments between the two, more so in rerecession. This can be avoided by engaging the upper border of LR first.

7.2.1.3 Inferior and Superior Recti Muscles

On both medial and lateral sides of the muscles, a vortex vein can be identified. Care must be taken as to not injure these veins during muscle handling. A complex fascial sheath system is present around the vertical recti attaching them to the respective lids and the obliques. Recessions of magnitude more than 5 mm may lead to lid retraction if good dissection is not done. The muscle should be adequately freed from the surrounding fascia to prevent this. The superior rectus (SR) muscle should be approached from the superotemporal quadrant and hooked near the insertion in order to avoid the superior oblique (SO) tendon from being engaged accidentally. In SR recessions, it is important to avoid suturing the muscle over the insertion of the SO. For this reason a hang-back procedure may be required for large SR recessions.

7.2.2 The Obliques

7.2.2.1 Superior Oblique Tendon
The anterior fibres of superior oblique (SO) are involved in intorsion of the globe, while the posterior fibres are selective for causing depression and abduction. The SO tendon is identified by its typical pearly white appearance. Its fan-shaped insertion is approached from the superotemporal side, whereas its chord portion is present nasal to the SR. Tuck (plication) procedure is not done superonasally as it may cause iatrogenic Brown syndrome.

7.2.2.2 Inferior Oblique Muscle
The inferior oblique (IO) is inserted temporally beneath the inferior border of the LR (Fig. 7.3). It is the only muscle that does not have a distal tendinous portion. It is distinctly identified by its dirty brown appearance in the Tenon's capsule unlike other muscles that are seen passing over the scleral surface. Due to its transverse course in the orbit, there is no risk of losing the muscle in the orbit. Anteriorisation of the IO weakens its action. IO should be carefully disinserted from the sclera as macula lies in its close proximity.

Fig. 7.3 The course of inferior oblique muscle

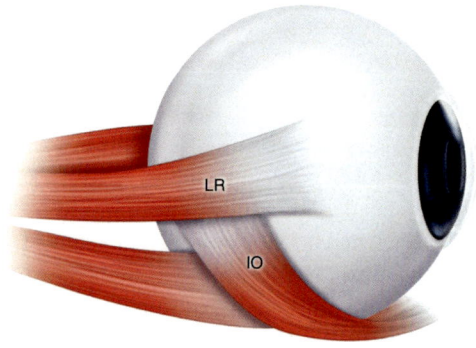

7.3   Physiological Considerations

An understanding of the physiological basis of action of the extraocular muscles is essential for obtaining foreseen surgical outcome. This mechanics of ocular movement is based on the relative innervational inputs to the muscles and also on the conversion of the linear power of the muscles into torque to rotate the globe in any of the *Listing's plane* [4]. The following determine the mechanics of ocular movements:

1. Strength and tightness of the muscle, i.e. torque generated to rotate the eye is directly proportional to the amount of contraction the muscle undergoes which in turn depends on the innervations of the muscle. In case of a paresis, the strength of the muscle is grossly decreased. Thus, as a strengthening procedure, mechanical shortening of the muscle tendon (resection) may be done on the paretic muscle to compensate for the decreased innervation. Similarly, an overacting muscle is weakened by lengthening its tendon (hang-back) or placing the insertion closer to origin (recession).
2. Length of the lever arm: The torque generated by a rectus muscle to rotate the globe depends on the leverage between the centre of rotation of the globe and the direction of pull of the muscle at point of contact. The more posterior this point of contact the shorter will be the lever arm and thus lower will be the torque generated. This principle is used to weaken a muscle's action in a selected gaze by a posterior fixation suture (Faden procedure also discussed in next chapter) (Fig. 7.4).

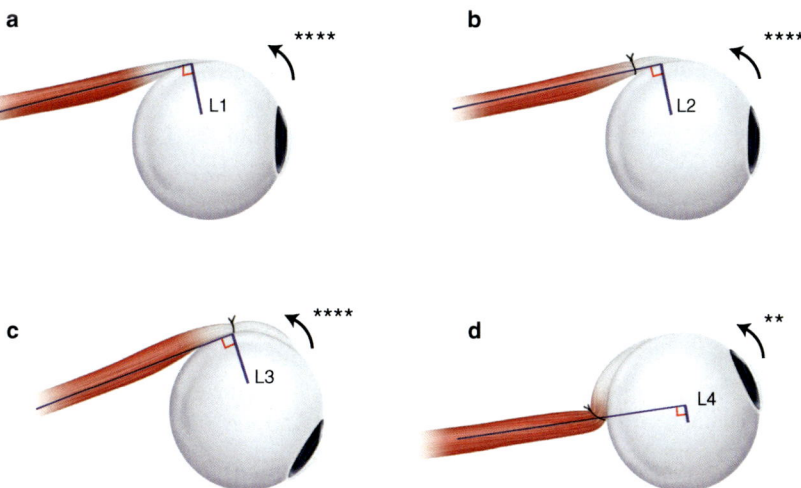

Fig. 7.4 Effect of Posterior Fixation suture (**a**) Normal lever arm L1; (**b** and **c**) after posterior fixation suture the lever arm L2 & L3 are unchanged in primary position and when the eye looks in opposite direction i.e. the muscle relaxes; (**d**) however it is significantly shortened L4 (generating lesser torque) when the muscle contracts

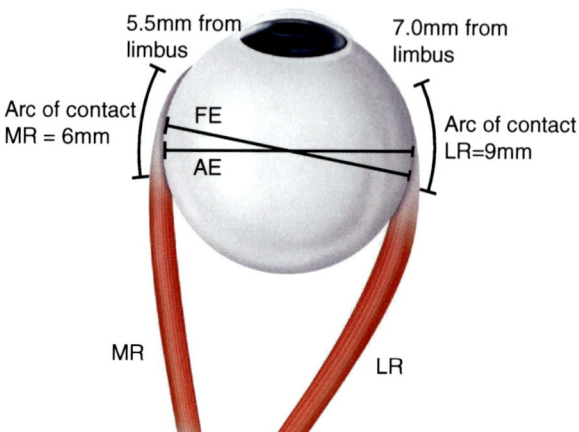

Fig. 7.5 Diagram showing anatomical equator (AE), functional equator (FE), arc of contact of medial rectus (MR) and lateral rectus (LR)

3. Arc of contact of the muscle: the medial and lateral recti run a course parallel to the medial and lateral orbital walls; thus the lateral rectus is longer than medial rectus. The axis of the globe is at 23° from the axis of the orbit. Thus the lateral rectus needs to curve around a larger area of the eyeball to reach its insertion, thereby having a longer length of muscle in contact with the eyeball. The longer arc of contact of the lateral rectus makes its lever arm shorter. The arc of contact decides the maximum amount of recession a muscle can undergo. The central point of arc of contact of the medial rectus lies anterior to the anatomical equator of the eye, whereas that of lateral rectus lies posterior to it (~2 mm). Line joining these points is the functional equator of the eyeball (Fig. 7.5). It is this functional equator which actually acts as the fulcrum for muscle action. Recession of a muscle beyond the line of functional equator will lead to loss of the action of the muscle leaving it only as a retractor muscle. From this discussion, it can be easily deduced that amount of maximal recession for the medial rectus is much less than that for lateral rectus muscle, i.e. about 7 mm and 10–12 mm, respectively. The actual position of the equator has been calculated from axial length and corneal diameter although its clinical utility has not been clearly established [5, 6]. But, it is proven that same amount of recession of the medial rectus will lead to a larger decrease in force of muscle action compared to lateral rectus.
4. The maximum amount of resection performed is 8 mm for MR and 10 mm for LR. It is limited to about 25% of the combined length of muscle and tendon to preserve muscle functionality.

7.4   Indications for Strabismus Surgery

Strabismus surgery is done for the following conditions.

1. To correct the static angle (Chap. 3) in comitant strabismus.
2. For correcting troublesome diplopia or anomalous head posture (AHP) in incomitant strabismus. This is usually achieved by restoring binocular single vision in *practical field of fixation* defined as the *area allowing central fixation by moving both eyes and head*, as in casual seeing [4]. Surgical management in incomitant deviations is considered after stabilisation of the etiology.
3. For correcting AHP and palpebral fissure abnormalities in restrictive conditions like Duane syndrome(Chap. 5).
4. In nystagmus to either shift the null point to primary position or to increase the effort of convergence in nystagmus blockage syndrome (Chap. 5).
5. For "cosmetic" alignment in sensory deviations. The alignment is more than cosmetic as strabismus has a significant psychosocial impact [7–9].

7.5   Determining "Target Angle" for Surgical Correction

Determination of the angle of squint has been discussed in Chap. 2. It has also been emphasised at several places that only the static angle of the squint should be corrected surgically. The following tests should be done to reveal the actual angle that needs to be corrected surgically.

1. *Patch test* is done in patients with near-distance disparity in the angle of deviation to eliminate the component of fusional convergence. Either eye of the patient is patched for 30–60 min [10]. Near deviation is remeasured immediately after removing the patch, taking care not to allow even a momentary binocular stimulation that could make the patient control the near deviation. This test differentiates simulated-divergence excess XT from true divergence excess XT (Chap. 3).
2. *+3.00 D spherical lens test* is done to determine the effect of accommodative convergence on near deviation. This test determines the AC/A ratio by gradient method as described in Chap. 3 and is essential in accommodative ET, as only the non-accommodative component of strabismus should be surgically corrected.
3. *Prism adaptation test (PAT)*: In all patients where postoperative binocularity is expected, a prism adaptation test should be done to determine the surgical dosage and predict the possibility of intractable diplopia after surgery. A trial of prisms to align the visual axes is given preoperatively. This stimulates restoration of fusion and predicts the potential of regaining binocular single vision. The largest prism with which the patient has binocular vision (and increasing prism causes diplopia) can be taken as the target angle for surgery.

In some patients the deviation may reappear after using the prism for some time. Then the deviation may be neutralised by a prism of larger magnitude. This process may occur in succession for a few prisms. This is known as "prism eating" or prism adaptation as after wearing the prisms, the patients return with a greater angle of deviation [11]. The patient is re-examined every 1–2 weeks and given larger prisms until the deviation stabilises [12]. The magnitude of the largest prism adapted angle is taken up for effective surgical correction [11, 13, 14].

7.6   Selection of Eye and the Muscle(s)

The selection of the eye to be operated upon is multifactorial. Preoperative binocular functions, visual acuity, ocular dominance (explained in Chap. 1), preference for fixation in primary gaze, presence of incomitance and parents' consent are the main points to be considered while planning surgery. In cases of large difference in visual acuity between the two eyes, usually the eye with the poorer vision has the deviation and is operated upon. But this decision is not always so straightforward.

Simplified guidelines for deciding the eye to be operated are given in the Table 7.3. However, it must be kept in mind that these are not absolute and should be interpreted with caution. Decision-making in strabismus, like in any other medical speciality, has to be individualized, and no set guidelines can be appropriate for all cases. In alternators with no preference to either eye, a bilateral surgery may be planned. In case of minimal difference in the visual acuity of the two eyes, the non-dominant eye is preferred to be taken up for surgery. Young children in whom binocular functions cannot be assessed are operated on lines of demonstrable binocularity (in Table 7.3) as they have often a good potential for binocular recovery.

Table 7.3 Deciding the eye to be operated

• *Demonstrable binocularity preoperatively*
– Bilateral symmetrical surgery or eye with better vision (non-dominant eye if similar vision)
• *No preoperative binocularity*
– Eye with worse vision
• *Paresis*
– Primary deviation (eye with paresis) if sound eye is fixating and secondary deviation (non-paretic eye) if patient fixes with the involved eye
• *Complete palsy*
– Muscle transposition in the eye with palsy or surgery on non-paralysed muscles in either eye
• *Restrictive component*
– Relieve the restriction as first step then reassess

Decision-making in different types of comitant and incomitant deviations has been discussed in Chaps. 2–4. The reader is reminded not to miss A/V patterns and oblique muscle dysfunctions while dealing with horizontal comitant deviations. While dealing with incomitant strabismus, it is imperative to distinguish paralytic component from restrictive as the surgical plan varies significantly. Surgery should be considered in paralytic deviations only when the etiology has been identified and the condition has been stable for at least 6 months. Hess charting, forced duction test (FDT) and force generation test (FGT) are essential for treatment planning in incomitant deviations. The most overacting muscle on Hess chart should be weakened. If restriction is confirmed on FDT, it should be released as a first step. Resection of a muscle with complete paralysis would have no effect.

7.6.1   Forced Duction Test (FDT)

This test is the most useful to rule out the presence of a restrictive component to strabismus. The conjunctiva is first anaesthetised with 4% xylocaine drops. A cotton swab wet with the anaesthetic may be additionally placed at the limbus where the globe will be held. A self-retaining speculum is applied, and the patient is instructed to look as far as possible in the direction of suspected limited duction. The globe is then passively forced into the direction opposite to where the restriction is suspected. For example, a long-standing esotropia may have some restriction of abduction due to a either a tight medial rectus (MR) or tight fascia (Text Box 7.1). In such a case, FDT is done by asking the patient to keep the involved eye in abduction (in order to relax the MR being tested). The examiner then holds the globe from the limbus near MR and pushes it in further abduction. In case of a restriction medially, the examiner will fail to do so or might feel resistance in doing so (positive FDT), whereas if the esotropia is only because of an underacting lateral rectus (LR), the examiner will be able to force the globe into full abduction. When being performed for the recti, the globe should be lifted up in order to keep the muscles stretched and pushed back when testing the obliques (exaggerated traction test—Text Box 7.2) [15].

This test is diagnostic of restrictive strabismus. In case of a positive result, releasing of the restrictive component is essential as a first step to align the eye. Subsequent surgery should be done after seeing its effect as releasing a tight muscle/tissue often causes an unpredictable (usually large) correction.

7.6.2   Force Generation Test (FGT)

FGT is an active test which helps differentiate a paresis from a complete paralysis. Although several techniques have been described, we recommend the one in which the FGT can be done in continuation of FDT [16]. In the example above where

Text Box 7.1: FDT and FGT for Esotropia

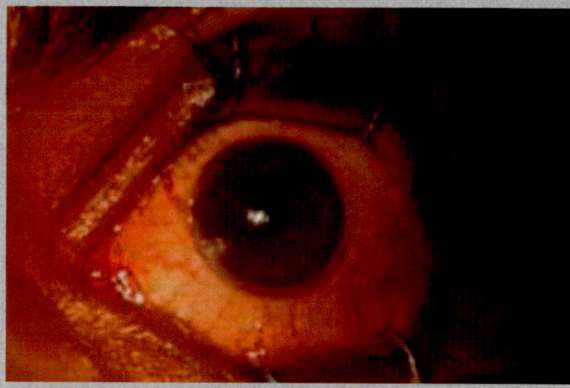

Step 1: After instillation of topical anaesthesia, the patient is asked to maximally abduct the eye.

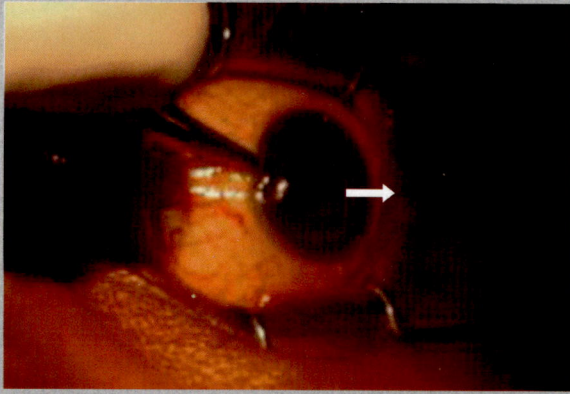

Step 2: Then the examiner firmly grasps the globe near the limbus and attempts to further abduct the eye and feel for resistance in *medial rectus* (FDT).

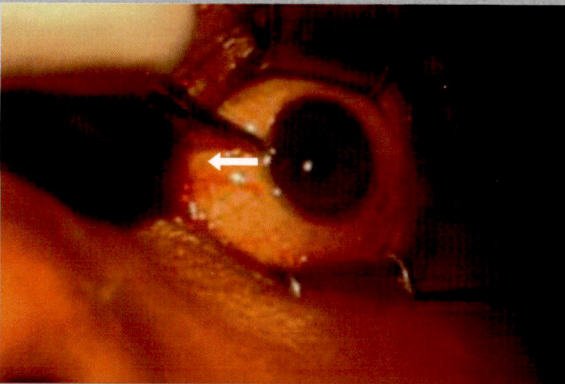

Step 3: The examiner then tries to adduct the eye while the patient is again asked to abduct. The examiner feels for a tug (or resistance) from the contracting *lateral rectus* (FGT).

Text Box 7.2: FDT for Superior Oblique

Step 1: The patient is asked to look up and in. The globe is held inferonasally and superotemporally at limbus.

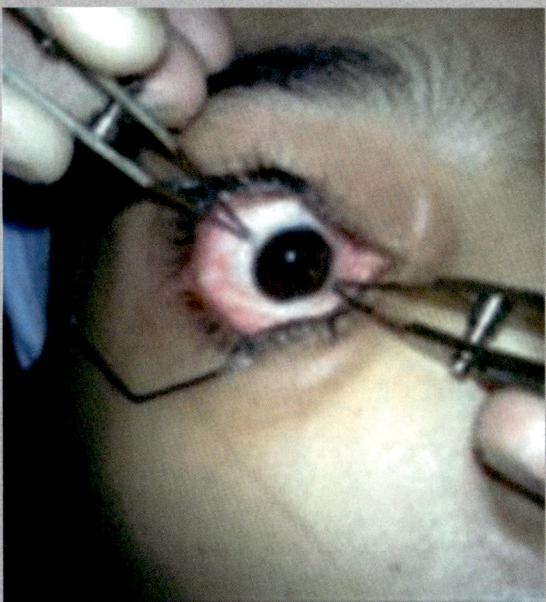

Step 2: Globe is then pushed in the orbit as it is elevated, adducted and rocked by extorting and intorting. Tautness of the tendon may be felt in extortion.

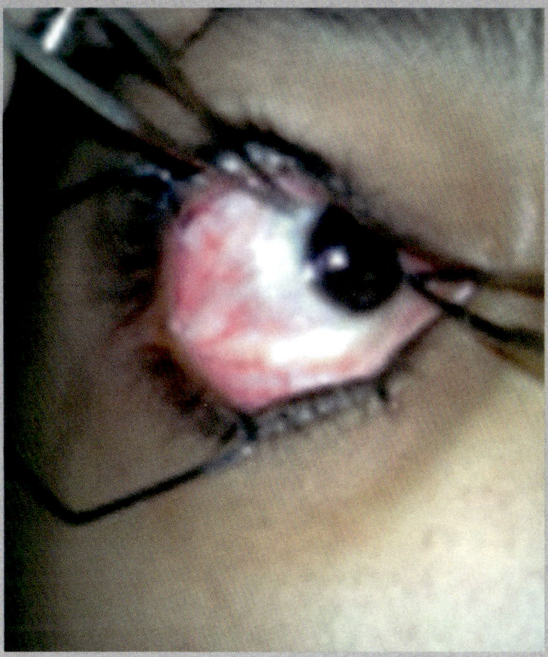

FDT was being done for MR, FGT would be indicated for LR to confirm its paresis or complete paralysis. So, after completion of FDT before releasing the forceps, the patient is again asked to maximally abduct his eye, while the examiner tries to adduct it (from holding it at the same point on limbus near MR) and evaluates the resistance (Text Box 7.1). If resistance is felt, it can be inferred that there is still some force being generated by the muscle, i.e. the muscle has paresis (positive FGT), and a strengthening procedure is likely to work. However, if no resistance is felt by the examiner, the muscle is paralysed and a transposition procedure would be needed.

7.7   Dosage of Surgery

Surgical dosage is amongst the most debated topics in strabismus. The presence of several tables and calculation methods is evidence that many lesser understood factors play a role in eventual surgical effect [17, 18]. Fortunately, there is consensus about several important points related to comitant deviations.

1. Recession plays a major part in restoration of ocular alignment, and resection has an accessory role [6, 18, 19].
2. Order of effectivity of horizontal muscle surgery is MR recession > LR recession > LR resection > MR recession [16, 20].
3. Correction for same surgery is larger in children than adults [16, 17, 21].
4. Correction is more in larger deviations [18, 20, 22].
5. Lesser correction per millimetre of surgery is achieved in larger eyes (greater axial length) [6, 23, 24].
6. Minimum recession recommended is about 3 mm for MR (2.5 mm in infants) and 5 mm for LR. The maximum recession that can be safely done is 7–8 mm of MR and up to 12 mm of LR [17, 22].
7. Minimum recommendation for resection is 3–4 mm for both horizontal recti. The maximum is 7–8 mm for MR and 10 mm for LR [17, 22].
8. Recession and resection surgery on one eye is more effective (about 25%) if performed together rather than in different sittings [25].
9. Motor outcome is better in presence of good binocular functions [1].
10. Each surgeon must record his results and try to develop his own dosage modifications [23, 26].
11. Desirable outcome in X(T) is slight overcorrection (6–10Δ) except in small children who should be orthotropic or under corrected [27–31].
12. Orthotropia is ideal, and microtropia (see Chap. 3) is an acceptable outcome for infantile ET [32].
13. Small ET should be aimed for, in all sensory tropias and patients with poor binocular functions.

Our dosage recommendations given in the Text Box 7.3 should be interpreted keeping the above factors in mind.

Text Box 7.3: Surgical Dosage

Range of expected correction in PD$^\Delta$ per mm of surgery in horizontal comitant deviations

MR rec	>	LR rec	>	LR res	>	MR res
5–3		4–2		3–1		2–1

Higher correction is achieved in presence of following (listed in decreasing order of priority)

- Deviation > 30$^\Delta$
- Age < 3 years
- Recession and resection being done together
- Axial length < 24 mm
- Recent onset

Equally important is the *surgeon's factor*. Neat dissection of muscle, severing surrounding attachments, minimal tissue trauma and appropriate closure would enhance the correction.

For example, a 15-year-old with a long-standing–40$^\Delta$ XT, axial length of 22 mm and a postoperative target of +5$^\Delta$ ET would require a bilateral LR recession of 7.5 mm considering a correction of 3$^\Delta$ per mm of surgery. The second option would be 10 mm LR recession with 7 mm MR resection (considering 3.5$^\Delta$ per mm of LR recession and 1.75$^\Delta$ per mm of MR resection) expecting a correction of about 43$^\Delta$.

7.8   Counselling Before Surgery

For a surgeon a satisfied patient is more important than a theoretically successful outcome. The most important factor in ensuring a satisfied patient is transparent management of expectations of the patient and his family members. The surgeon must explain the condition, the treatment options and the expected outcome. The patient or parents must be involved in decision-making. A detailed informed consent must be obtained. It is of utmost importance that expectations from the surgery are realistic else a successful outcome for the surgeon might be perceived as a failure by the patient and his family.

7.9   Summary

- Understanding anatomic and physiologic factors which determine the mechanics of ocular movements is essential for meticulous surgical planning of strabismus.
- The torque generated to rotate the eyeball depends upon the muscle innervation and muscle centration.
- The muscle strength, lever arm and arc of contact of muscle are important determinants of ocular movement mechanics.
- While planning surgical correction, target angle of surgical correction should be ascertained using patch or prism adaptation test to avoid suboptimal correction.

- Surgical correction in comitant strabismus is usually done on the non-dominant eye or the eye with poor vision.
- FDT is useful to differentiate between paralytic and restrictive strabismus.
- Restriction should be relieved before planning definitive surgical correction.
- Muscle transposition surgery should be planned in presence of complete paralysis of extraocular muscles.
- The surgical dose for strabismus correction may vary depending upon operating surgeon. However, for horizontal muscles, recession surgeries are more effective on MR and resection on LR.
- Patient counselling and projecting realistic postoperative expectations are important considerations in surgical planning of strabismus.

7.10 Multiple Choice Questions

1. The maximum amount of recession a muscle can undergo depends upon
   (a) Length of its tendinous part
   (b) Arc of contact of muscle
   (c) Distance of muscle from limbus
   (d) All of the above

Answer: (b) The maximum amount of recession a muscle can undergo is decided by its arc of contact with the globe. If a muscle is recessed beyond its arc of contact, it may lose its action.

2. Faden procedure on medial rectus will have a maximum effect on which of the following?
   (a) Primary position of eyeball
   (b) Abduction
   (c) Convergence
   (d) None of the above

Answer: (c) Faden procedure selectively weakens a muscle in the direction of its action because the lever arm of the muscle is almost unchanged in primary position, but as the eye moves in the field of action of muscle, the lever arm is substantially shortened. Of all of the above, medial rectus acts during convergence.

3. Which of the following muscle has no risk of being lost in orbit during surgery?
   (a) Lateral rectus
   (b) Inferior rectus
   (c) Inferior oblique
   (d) Superior oblique

Answer: (c) Inferior oblique due to its transverse course in the orbit has no risk of being lost in the orbit.

4. A patient of exotropia was found to have limitation of ocular movement in adduction. On performing forced duction test, the eye could not be adducted fully. Which of the following statements is true regarding management of this patient?
   (a) There is medial rectus restriction, so medial rectus recession should be considered.
   (b) There is lateral rectus muscle restriction, so lateral rectus recession should be considered.
   (c) There is medial rectus muscle palsy, so medial rectus resection should be done.
   (d) There is lateral rectus muscle palsy, so lateral rectus resection should be planned.

Answer: (b) The FDT is positive for lateral rectus muscle in this case, which implies that there is restriction due to lateral rectus muscle. Releasing the restrictive component is essential as an initial step to align the eye. Subsequent surgery should be done after seeing its effect as releasing a tight muscle/tissue often causes an unpredictable (usually large) correction.

5. The following statements are true regarding resection of muscle *except*:
   (a) It is a strengthening procedure.
   (b) There is no limit to maximum resection of a muscle.
   (c) The minimum recommended resection for horizontal recti is 3–4 mm.
   (d) None of the above.

Answer: (b) The maximum amount of resection performed is 8 mm for MR and 10 mm for LR. It is limited to about 25% of the combined length of muscle and tendon to preserve muscle functionality.

References

1. Singh V, Pandey M, Agrawal S. Binocular potential score: a novel concept. J Pediatr Ophthalmol Strabismus. 2008;45(2):104–8.
2. Plager DA, Parks MM. Recognition and repair of the slipped rectus muscle. J Pediatr Ophthalmol Strabismus. 1988;25:270–4.
3. Chatzistefanou KI, Kushner BJ, Gentry LR. Magnetic resonance imaging of the arc of contact of extraocular muscles: implications regarding the incidence of slipped muscles. J AAPOS. 2000;4(2):84–93.
4. Von Noorden GK, Campos EC. Chapter 4: Physiology of the ocular movements. In: Binocular vision and ocular motility. 6th ed. St. Louis: Mosby; 2002. p. 52–84.
5. Kuscher BJ, Fisher MR, Lucchese NJ, Morton GV. How far can medial rectus safely be recessed? J Pediatr Ophthalmol Strabismus. 1994;31:138.
6. Kuscher BJ, Fisher MR, Lucchese NJ, Morton GV. Factors influencing response to strabismus surgery. Arch Ophthalmol. 1993;111:75.
7. Durnian JM, Noonan CP, Marsh IB. The psychosocial effects of adult strabismus: a review. Br J Ophthalmol. 2011;95:450–3.
8. Olitsky SE, Sudesh S, Graziano A, Hamblen J, Brooks SE, Shaha SH. The negative psychosocial impact of strabismus in adults. J AAPOS. 1999;3(4):209–11.
9. Mojon-Azzi SM, Kunz A, Mojon DS. Strabismus and discrimination in children: are children with strabismus invited to fewer birthday parties? Br J Ophthalmol. 2011;95:473–6.

10. Wright KW, Spiegel PH, Thompson LS. Chapter 8: Exotropia. In: Handbook of pediatric strabismus and amblyopia. NY: Springer; 2006. p. 270–1.
11. Herzau V, Schoser G. The value of the prism adaptation test in determining the degree of squint surgery. Ophthalmologe. 1993;90(1):11–6.
12. Repka MX, Connett JE, Scott WE. The one-year surgical outcome after prism adaptation for the management of acquired esotropia. Ophthalmology. 1996;103(6):922–8.
13. Dadeya S, Kamlesh, Naniwal S. Usefulness of the preoperative prism adaptation test in patients with intermittent exotropia. J Pediatr Ophthalmol Strabismus. 2003;40(2):85–9.
14. Schildwächter-von Langenthal A, Kommerell G, Klein U, Simonsz HJ. Preoperative prism adaptation test in normosensoric strabismus. Graefes Arch Clin Exp Ophthalmol. 1989;227(3):206–8.
15. Guyton D. Exaggerated traction test for oblique muscles. Ophthalmology. 1981;88:1035.
16. Rosenbaum AL, Urrea PT. Investigation of limited ocular rotations: current status. Am Orthopt J. 1987;37:1.
17. Rosenbaum AL, Santiago AP. Surgical dose tables. In: Clinical strabismus management principles and surgical techniques. Philadelphia, PA: WB Saunders Company; 2001. p. 553.
18. von Noorden GK, Campos EC. Principles of surgical treatment. In: Binocular vision and ocular motility: theory and management of strabismus. 6th ed. St. Louis, MO: CV Mosby; 2001. p. 571–3.
19. Kushner BJ. How do recessions and resections of extraocular muscles work? J AAPOS. 2006;10:291–2.
20. Yurdakul NS, Bodur S, Koç F. Surgical results of symmetric and asymmetric surgeries and dose-response in patients with infantile esotropia. Turk J Ophthalmol. 2015;45(5):197–202.
21. Abbasoglu OE, Sener EC, Sanac AS. Factors influencing the successful outcomeand response in strabismus surgery. Eye. 1996;10:315–20.
22. Umazume F, Ohtsuki H, Hasebe S. Preoperative factors influencing effectiveness of surgery in adult strabismus. Jpn J Ophthalmol. 1997;41(2):89–97.
23. Rosenbaum AL, Santiago AP. Factors influencing measurement and response to strabismus surgery. In: Clinical strabismus management principles and surgical techniques. Philadelphia, PA: WB Saunders Company; 2001. p. 77.
24. Agrawal S, Singh V, Gupta SK, Agrawal S. Evaluating a new surgical dosage calculation method for esotropia. Oman J Ophthalmol. 2013;6:165–9.
25. Roper-Hall MJ. The extraocular muscles: strabismus and heterophoria. In: Stallard's eye surgery. 7th ed. London: Wright; 1989. p. 169–70.
26. Kushner BJ, Preslan MW, Vrabec M. Artifacts of measuring during strabismus surgery. J Pediatr Ophthalmol Strabismus. 1987;24(4):159–64.
27. McNeer KW. Observations on the surgical overcorrection of childhood intermittent exotropia. Am Orthopt J. 1987;37:135–50.
28. Raab EL, Parks MM. Recession of the lateral recti. Arch Ophthalmol. 1969;82:203–8.
29. Scott WE, Keech R, Mash AJ. The post-operative results and stability of exodeviations. Arch Ophthalmol. 1981;99(10):1814–8.
30. Souza-Dias C, Uesugi CF. Post-operative evolution of the planned initial over-correction in intermittent exotropia: 61 cases. Binocul Vis Eye Muscle Surg Q. 1993;1003:141–8.
31. Raab EC. Management of Intermittent exotropia : for surgery. Am Orthopt J. 1998;48:25–9.
32. von Noorden GK, Campos EC. Chapter 16: Esodeviations. In: Binocular vision and ocular motility. 6th ed. St. Louis: Mosby; 2002. p. 311–49.

Horizontal Muscle Strabismus Surgery

8

Siddharth Agrawal, Priyanka Singh,
and Rajat M. Srivastava

8.1 Introduction

Surgical success is determined by precision in execution of the surgical process, which in turn depends on clear understanding of the technique. This chapter will highlight the instrumentation, anesthesia, and surgical techniques of horizontal muscle strabismus surgery.

8.2 Operating Microscope

Ideally, all strabismus surgeries should be performed under operating microscope. Magnified and clear visualization of the extraocular muscles (EOM) and their fascia is essential for clean surgical dissection and precise measurements. Magnification loupe may be used as an inferior alternative.

8.3 Instrumentation

The instruments used in strabismus surgery are shown in Fig. 8.1. A self-retaining speculum is preferred for adequate exposure. There are a variety of muscle hooks, but ones with shoulder (Jamesons or Green) should be used by beginners as they resist the slipping out of the muscle from the hook during manipulations.

The commonly used sutures are depicted in the photograph. 6-0 silk on spatulated needle is used for fixation of the globe at 12 and 6 o'clock positions for

S. Agrawal (✉) · R. M. Srivastava
Department of Ophthalmology, King George's Medical University, Lucknow, India

P. Singh
Aravind Eye Hospital, Madurai, India

© Springer Nature Singapore Pte Ltd. 2019
S. Agrawal (ed.), *Strabismus*, https://doi.org/10.1007/978-981-13-1126-0_8

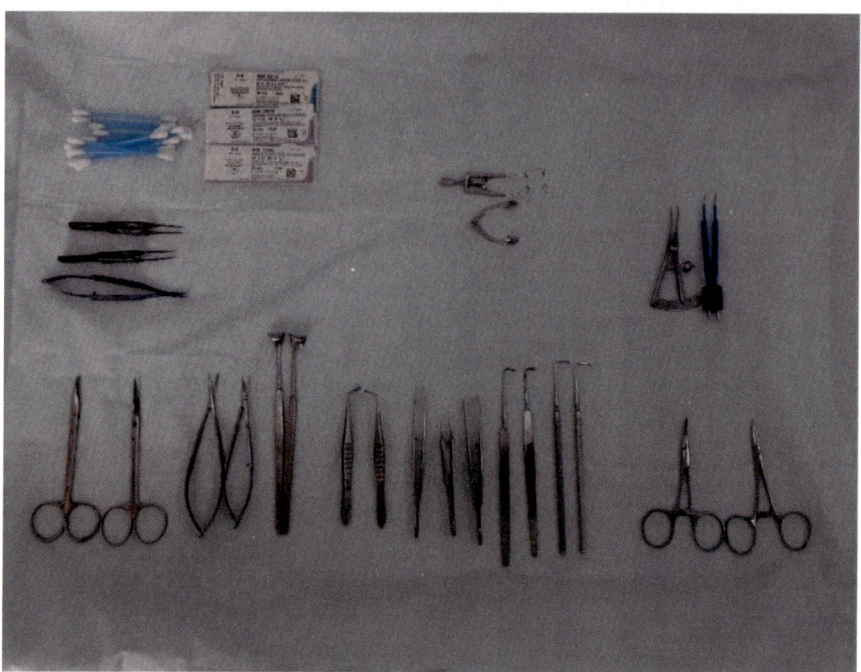

Fig. 8.1 Strabismus trolley. Clockwise from top left. Sterile mops, sutures: coated vicryl (poly-glactin 910) 6-0 (on spatulated needle like S-29), vicryl 8-0 and silk 6-0 (on spatulated needle like S-14), self-retaining speculum (adult and pediatric), calipers (Castroviejo), bipolar forceps, mosquito hemostats-2, muscle hooks (Green-2 and Graefe-2), forceps (Prince muscle, Pierse Hoskins and Wills Hospital utility-1 each), muscle clamp (Jamesons-2), Desmarres retractors-2, Westcott conjunctival scissors-2, Steven's tenotomy scissors (curved and straight), needle holder (Castroviejo), and suturing forceps (Castroviejo—straight and curved)

horizontal muscle surgeries. 6-0 silk on round needle may also be used as a marking suture for identification of the edges of the conjunctival incision (explained later). The muscles are sutured with 6-0 polyglactin (vicryl) on S-14 or S-29 spatulated needle. Conjunctival incision can be closed with either 8-0 or 9-0 vicryl with buried knots or with fibrin glue. The latter has advantages of being faster, having better cosmesis and lesser foreign body sensation postoperatively.

Thus, squint surgery can be performed in any general ophthalmology setup with minimal additional instrumentation.

8.4   Choice of Anesthesia

This decision has to be individualized depending on the age of the patient, his level of cooperation, willingness to tolerate some discomfort, surgeon's skills, and the procedure being considered. However certain points must be kept in mind.

1. General anesthesia (GA) should be used in all children <12 years and in uncooperative patients. It should also be considered in adults desiring the least possible discomfort after discussion of pros and cons. Depolarizing muscle relaxants (suxamethonium) should be avoided till forced duction test (FDT) is performed as they cause prolonged extraocular muscle relaxation.
2. Local anesthesia is provided with a combination of varying amounts of 1–2% lignocaine and 0.5% bupivacaine. The routes of administration are:
   (a) Retrobulbar injection provides orbital anesthesia and akinesia. It also blocks the potential oculocardiac reflex and does not need a facial nerve block. It should however be performed by an individual well versed in the technique and avoided in high myopes due to potential sight-threatening complication of globe penetration [1].
   (b) Peribulbar injection has significantly lesser incidence of globe injury [2], but it takes longer time to achieve complete effect and often requires more than one injection. This is our preferred technique of local anesthesia.
   (c) Sub-Tenon's injection after anesthetizing the cul-de-sac with 0.5% proparacaine hydrochloride is an effective method. The anesthetic agent is injected in sub-Tenon's space 3 mm from the limbus, anterior to the muscle insertion. It is safe, has faster onset, and does not affect optic nerve function.
3. Topical anesthesia is achieved in consenting adults by frequent drops of 0.5% proparacaine hydrochloride, similar to cataract surgery. Though initially used for postoperative adjustments in adjustable suture technique, we and many others perform recessions in cooperative patients under topical anesthesia [3]. The complications associated with injection anesthesia are avoided with the added advantage of being able to adjust sutures on table with greater accuracy. Topical anesthesia is not recommended in initial cases of the surgeon.
4. Topical diluted adrenaline (epinephrine) or brimonidine may be used to reduce intraoperative bleeding [4].
5. Risk of oculocardiac reflex (OCR) due to vagal stimulation should always be kept in mind. The patient may complain of nausea if under local anesthesia. OCR is characterized by sinus bradycardia, nodal rhythm, ectopic beats, or sinus arrest during handling of extraocular muscles, especially medial rectus. Prompt diagnosis should be followed by immediate release of muscle. If it persists, intravenous atropine (0.15 mg/kg) is given. In recalcitrant cases, retrobulbar lignocaine is recommended to block the afferent loop. OCR is commoner in young children undergoing strabismus surgery under GA. It is advisable to have monitoring electrodes connected and have an anesthetist standby even in cases being performed under local anesthesia.

8.5   Horizontal Muscle Strabismus Surgery

Before embarking upon surgery, the patient's identity, surgical plan, and the eye to be operated should be confirmed by the surgeon himself. There can be no greater misfortune than to make a mistake in any of these which is a real possibility in a busy operation theater. FDT is done to rule out any restrictive component in all patients both before and after completion of surgery. In certain cases the surgical plan is decided or altered in the operating room itself after a FDT. In cases where this is a possibility, prior informed consent must be taken.

Cleaning with povidone iodine and draping are performed as usual.

8.5.1   Fixation Suture

A fixation suture is applied with 6-0 silk on spatulated needle at 12 and 6 o'clock close to limbus, through the conjunctiva and superficial sclera. The eye is rotated and fixed with these sutures to expose the site of surgery (rotated laterally for medial rectus surgery and medially for lateral rectus). The position of the fixation sutures is altered in vertical muscle surgeries.

Application of two fixation sutures helps in adequate exposure without inadvertently causing globe rotation. Globe rotation may misalign the anatomical landmarks and complicate the surgery. Locking forceps (e.g. Castroviejo) are better alternative to fixation sutures.

8.5.2   Conjunctival Incision

An ideal conjunctival incision should provide liberal exposure of EOM without compromising the cosmesis. Various conjunctival incisions have been described. Fornix incisions and minimally invasive strabismus surgery (MISS) [5] require significant expertise and should not be attempted by beginners. It has been demonstrated by others and us that the limbal incision is best suited for initial cases as it offers good exposure, minimal need for assistance, and acceptable cosmesis [6, 7]. The incision is extended radially by 3–4 mm at one or both ends (Fig. 8.2).

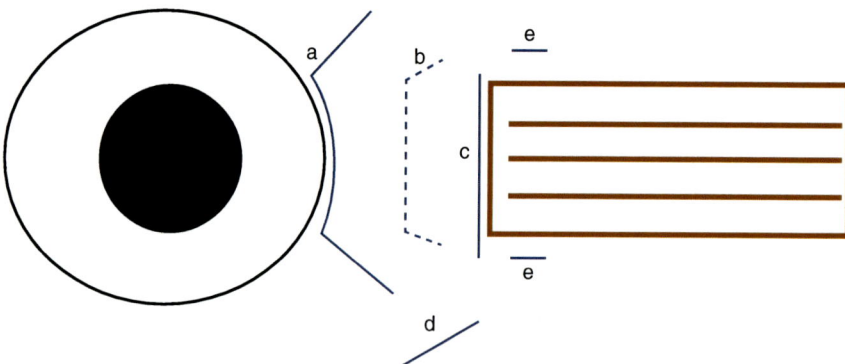

Fig. 8.2 Various incisions described for strabismus surgeries. (**a**) Limbal incision with radial extensions is recommended for beginners [6, 8], (**b**) midway between muscle and limbus [9], (**c**) near the insertion [10]. (**d**) Fornix incision used by experts gives better cosmesis [11], (**e**) two small incisions used in minimally invasive strabimus surgery (MISS) [5]

8.5.3   Exposure of the Muscle

The conjunctiva and Tenon's capsule are tightly adherent close to the limbus; thus the limbal incision provides entry to the sub-Tenon's space. Care must be taken not to dissect between the conjunctiva and Tenon's capsule. The combined layer of conjunctiva and Tenon's capsule is carefully separated from the episclera by dissection with blunt Westcott scissors. The conjunctiva (along with attached Tenon's capsule) is then retracted back after passing 6-0 silk suture at its edges, for easy identification at the time of closure (Fig. 8.3). The dissection to separate Tenon's capsule from episclera must not be done in the area where muscle insertion is expected, to avoid inadvertent injury to muscle fibers which may cause troublesome bleeding. An opening is made in intermuscular septa to reach bare sclera. Muscle hook is then passed by gentle sweeping, and any resistance in previously unoperated eye should make the surgeon suspicious of being in the wrong plane. The muscle hook is inserted with its tip pointing away from the insertion, and the muscle is engaged by rotating the hook 180°. The lower border of the muscle is engaged first. Traction on the handle of the hook exposes the muscle allowing intermuscular septa to be identified and freed by sharp dissection. Injury to the muscle sheath should be avoided. The second hook is then passed to expose the upper border of the muscle which is similarly exposed and dissected. The hooks should be gently swiped back to break any adhesions between muscle and sclera. The edge of the insertion should be checked to ensure that the complete muscle is engaged and no fibers are left. Accidental engagement of fibers of the inferior oblique may occur while isolating the lateral rectus muscle, more so during reoperations. This may be avoided by passing the first hook from above.

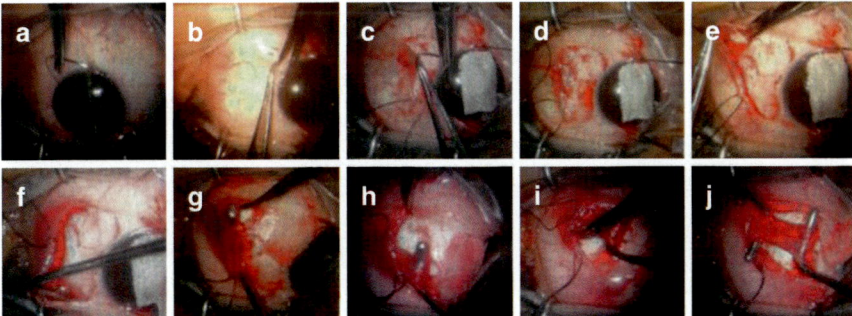

Fig. 8.3 Exposure of horizontal recti. (**a**) Traction suture at the limbus. (**b**) Limbal conjunctival incision with radial cuts perpendicular to limbus. (**c**) Conjunctival marking suture. (**d**) Conjunctiva and Tenon's capsule reflected. (**e**) Blunt dissection with Westcott scissors for separation of anterior Tenon's capsule and intermuscular septum dissection should not be done in the area where muscle insertion is expected, to avoid muscle injury. (**f**) Muscle hook is inserted below the muscle near its insertion with its tip pointing away from the insertion. (**g**) Muscle is engaged by rotating the hook and exposed by applying traction on the handle. (**h, i**) Freeing of the borders of the muscle from the facial connections and the conjunctival surface by sharp dissection. (**j**) Second hook is passed at the superior border, and the muscle is freed by dissection

The distance to which dissection is carried out (from the muscle insertion) is usually 6 mm for the medial rectus and 8 mm for the lateral rectus (may be a little more for resections).

8.5.4   Recession of Muscle

Recessions are the most commonly performed weakening procedure, where the muscle is disinserted and attached some distance behind the insertion. After exposure of muscle as discussed, bipolar wet field cautery is used at the muscle insertion followed by securing it with two separate single-armed 6-0 vicryl (with spatulated needle). Both superior and inferior ends of the muscle are secured, not more than 1 mm from insertion site (Fig. 8.4). Two bites are taken from each end, one involving full muscle belly and the other with partial thickness, carefully locking the suture at each end. Muscle is detached using Westcott scissor taking care not to cut sclera or suture. Desired amount of recession is marked using caliper from both the ends of the muscle stump. Castroviejo caliper is usually used for measurements; however, measuring along the curvature of the globe (the arc) is believed to be more accurate [12] (Fig. 8.5).

The ends of the muscle are attached at the marks taking care that the needle does not pass too deep into the sclera. The knots should not be too tight or loose.

> *Clinical Tip: While performing large recessions of lateral rectus, it should be kept in mind that macula lies beneath, and perforation while taking scleral bite can be disastrous!*

The usual range of recessions is from 3 to 7 mm for medial recti and 4 to 8 mm for lateral recti. Larger recessions may be performed in extremely large deviations,

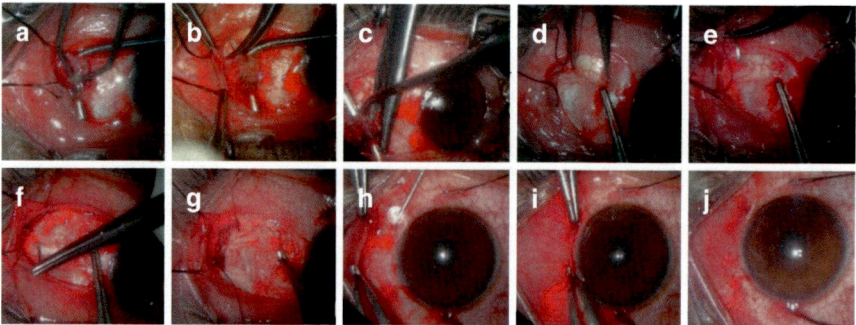

Fig. 8.4 Recession surgery of horizontal recti. (**a**) After the rectus muscle is engaged and cleared of its attachments, the insertion is cauterized. (**b**) The muscle is secured on two preplaced sutures behind the cauterized site. (**c**) The muscle is cut at the insertion. (**d**) Marking the site of recession on the sclera with caliper. (**f**) Taking scleral bite at the marked distance. (**g**) Securing the muscle to this new site. (**h–j**) Conjunctival closure using fibrin glue

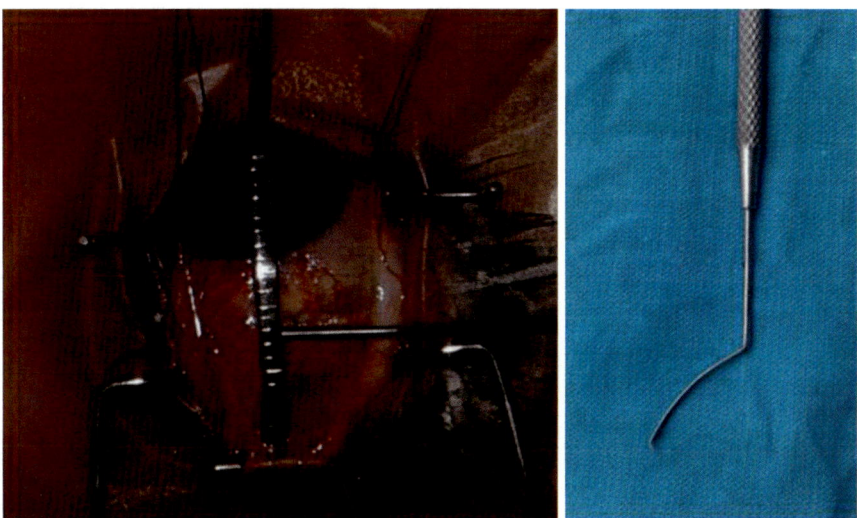

Fig. 8.5 Our self-designed caliper offers several advantages like being free from calibration errors, measuring the arc (and not the chord) and ease of holding. (Patent pending: Singh-Agrawal ruler, Temp/30105/2015-Del)

in myopic eyes, or with adjustable sutures. Greater caution is required in exceeding the limit (7 mm) with MR than with LR (which may be recessed up to 12 mm) as the functional equator is more anteriorly placed on the medial side. Troublesome limitation of adduction and convergence may occur if the medial rectus is recessed beyond the functional equator. The actual amount of surgery required depends on various factors discussed in the previous chapter.

8.5.4.1 Simple Modifications of Recession

In patients with thinned out sclera (myopia) and large recessions, one can use *hang-back* or *hemi-hang-back recessions*. For hang-back technique, the surgeon passes the two sutures (on which the detached muscle is secured) at the original insertion and ties a knot after allowing a slack in the suture to account for the recession distance (Fig. 8.6a). In hemi-hang back, the hang back is performed from a point posterior to the original insertion making it a combination of recession and hang back (Fig. 8.6b).

Similarly, *adjustable sutures* are used with bow tie/shoe lace knot or with a sliding noose (Fig. 8.6c) [13]. Adjustable sutures are known to improve the surgical success not only in patients with unpredictable outcomes such as paralytic strabismus, restrictive strabismus, thyroid ophthalmopathy, etc. but also in comitant deviations [14–17] (Text Box 8.1). We recommend that after gaining experience in initial cases, the surgeon should start doing adjustable recessions [17–19].

The modifications in steps from conventional recession are simple to follow (Figs. 8.6 and 8.7). The muscle is anchored on double armed 6-0 vicryl at both ends and the suture bites taken at the original insertion including the muscle stump and superficial sclera. A partial thickness scleral bite taken in the hang-back length is

Fig. 8.6 Simple modifications of recession. (**a**) Hang-back recession. (**b**) Hemi-hang-back recession. (**c**) Modified adjustable hang-back recession. (Legend 1, original muscle insertion; 2, adjustable length; 3, partial thickness sclera bite; 4, bow tie knot)

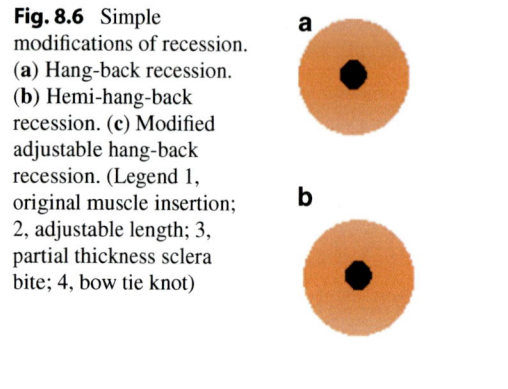
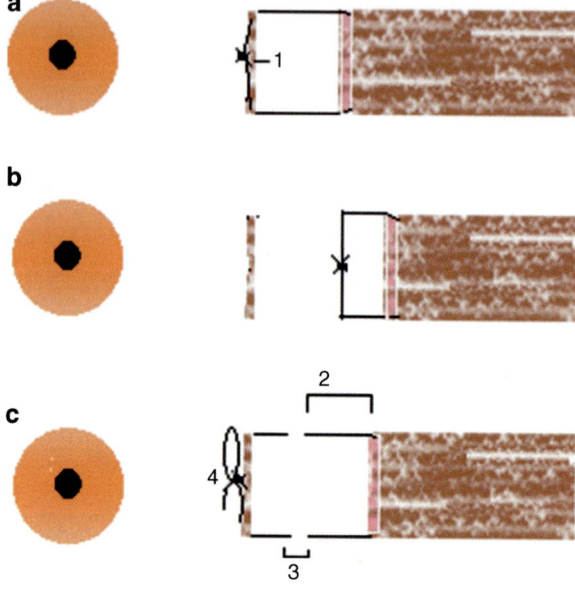

Text Box 8.1: Indications for Adjustable Sutures

Whenever the results of conventional surgery are unpredictable or greater accuracy is desirable.

- Reoperations
- Extremes of deviation (large for unpredictability and small for greater accuracy)
- Paralytic squints
- Restrictive or combined mechanism strabismus (thyroid eye disease, after trauma, or in presence of explants like buckles, glaucoma valves, etc.)

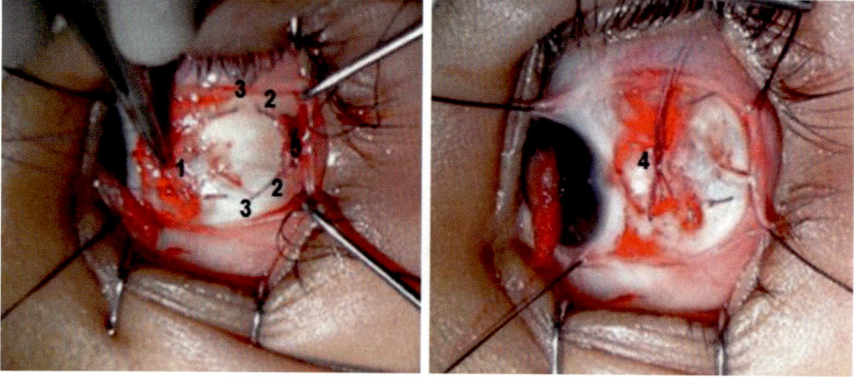

Fig. 8.7 Modified adjustable recession. (Legend 1, original muscle insertion; 2, adjustable length; 3, partial thickness sclera bite; 4, bow tie knot; 5, muscle anchored on double armed 6-0 vicryl)

Table 8.1 Preferred position of alignment at the time of adjustment [20]

Type of strabismus	Position of alignment (PD or Δ)
Exodeviations	+5 to +10 Δ
Esodeviations	
With fusion potential	0 to −5 Δ
Without fusion potential	+2 to +7 Δ

believed to improve outcomes. The muscle is then allowed to recede back a desired amount. The sutures should be moved back and forth a few times to widen the suture tunnels in sclera to enable easy adjustment later. The sutures are then tied in a double knot with the second knot being a bow knot. The end which will open the knot is left longer for identification. The conjunctiva is closed in usual manner. Should the sutures need adjustment (as per Table 8.1), the conjunctiva is opened under topical anesthesia, bow knot released, and the sutures pulled up. As pulling up of sutures is easier than pushing back, it is advisable to plan slight overcorrection with the option of pulling them up. The conjunctiva is repositioned with tissue glue or sutures in usual manner. The exact timing of adjustment is controversial with on table adjustment recommended for surgery under topical anesthesia to up to few weeks later [21, 22]. We prefer to do the adjustment on the third day to allow the edema to subside, making the procedure more comfortable for the patient. It also allows for early postoperative drift [21]. Also, we do not open the conjunctiva to retie the knots if the surgical outcome is satisfactory [17]. We, like many others, do not advocate adjustable resection [19, 23, 24].

Offset or slanting of insertions is done for correction of A and V patterns in the absence of oblique muscle dysfunction (Text Box 8.2).

Text Box 8.2: "A" & "V" Patterns

Identification and clinical significance of these patterns have been discussed in Chap. 5. Two simple modifications of recession-resection surgery enables their correction in the *absence of oblique muscle dysfunction*. In presence of latter, management of oblique dysfunction should be the treatment of choice.

Offset or displacement of insertions:

As a rule the medial rectus (MR) insertion is shifted toward the apex of the pattern, and lateral rectus (LR) is shifted toward the base. Thus, for a V pattern, displacement of MR would be down and of LR up. Reverse would be done for A pattern. Usually, a full tendon width (10 mm) displacement is done.

Slanting the insertions: Though less effective than offsets, this is easier to perform. The margin of the muscle where greater weakening is desired is recessed more. For example, in V pattern XT, the upper margin of LR is recessed more than the lower margin. Similarly, for greater effect of strengthening, the upper margin of MR is resected more.

Other weakening procedures are Faden operation (Text Box 8.3), free tenotomy, and marginal myotomy.

Text Box 8.3: Posterior Fixation Suture (Faden or Retroequatorial Myopexy). See Fig. 7.4

Principle: The action of a rectus muscle is selectively weakened in its primary field of action without disturbing the balance between agonist and antagonist in other positions of gaze.

Indications: Patients who require a gaze selective weakening like (a) paresis with diplopia in peripheral gaze and (b) nystagmus blockage syndrome (NBS).

Procedure: Yoke of the muscle with paresis or MR in NBS is attached to the sclera with a nonabsorbable suture beyond its functional equator (12–15 mm from original insertion).

8.5.5   Resection of Muscle

Resection is a strengthening procedure involving excision of a predetermined length of the muscle comprising primarily of the tendinous portion (starting from the insertion) and suturing the remaining muscle to the insertion, in effect tightening the muscle.

After isolating the muscle, the resection distance is marked with calipers (Fig. 8.8). Caution must be exercised in measurement by exerting minimal pull on the muscle as the measurement must be done on an unstretched muscle. Also, inadvertent plication of the muscle may occur during measurement, resulting in over-resection (Fig. 8.9). The muscle insertion and the point of resection are cauterized

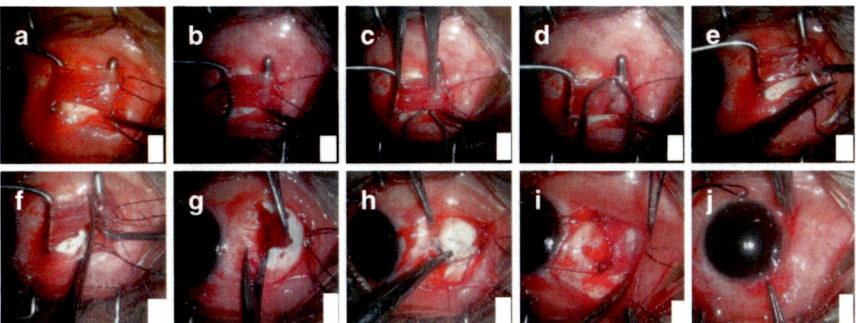

Fig. 8.8 Resection surgery of horizontal recti. (**a**) Engaging and clearing the muscle. (**b**) Insertion is cauterized. (**c**) Measuring the length of the muscle to be resected. (**d**) Cauterization at the marked site. (**e**) Preplacement of sutures behind the cauterized line. (**f, g**) Muscle stump cut and removed. (**h**) Securing the muscle to the original insertion site. (**i**) Pulling the cut muscle end up to the original insertion and cutting the sutures. (**j**) Closure of the conjunctiva

Fig. 8.9 Care should be taken while measuring, as excessive pull results in plication of the muscle below the hook (arrow) resulting in erroneous measurements

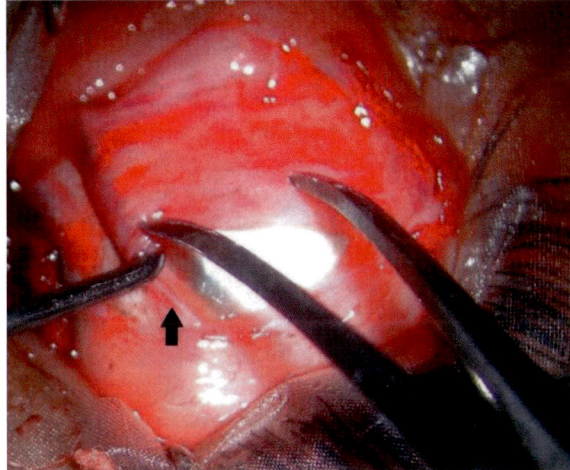

with a wet field bipolar cautery. Vicryl 6-0 suture is passed and secured at both borders of the muscle, proximal to the mark created by cautery. The extra muscle distal to the sutures is excised with Westcott scissors. Care should be taken not to cut too close to the sutures, lest the muscle may slip. On excision of muscle stump from insertion, some oozing may occur which may be controlled by pressure over the insertion. The limbal fixation sutures are released, and muscle is brought back and sutured to the insertion from where the stump has been detached. Superficial sclera should also be included in the suture bite along with the muscle stump to prevent muscle slippage later.

Text Box 8.4: Strabismus Surgeries
Weakening Procedures
- Recession
- Faden (retroequatorial myopexy)
- Marginal myotomy
- Tenotomy/myectomy or disinsertion
- Lengthening (by sutures or silicon expander)

Strengthening Procedures
- Resection
- Advancement
- Plication/double breasting
- Transposition

Common muscle transposition procedures have been discussed in Chap. 4.

Intermuscular attachments should be released by sharp dissection. For lateral rectus resections, it is important as mentioned earlier to severe it's attachment with inferior oblique else a resultant vertical deviation may result. In medial rectus resections, the anatomy of the plica should be preserved.

Usual range of resection is from 4 to 8 mm for MR and 4 to 10 mm for LR [6]. Where greater effect of resection is desirable or predetermined, amount of resection could not be done due to various reasons; augmentation may be done simply by *advancing* the insertion by 1–2 mm toward the limbus.

Von Noorden has described the use of muscle clamps and securing of the muscle with sutures after being detached from insertion for resection [6]. This, however, requires a larger incision and trained assistance.

Various strabismus surgeries have been listed in Text Box 8.4.

Clinical Tip: Medial rectus is more likely to slip and difficult to retrieve as it has a straighter course and has no attachments to the oblique muscles.

8.5.6 Conjunctival Closure

Conjunctiva is pulled back to the limbus with the help of the marking sutures and secured. The marking sutures are removed after the conjunctiva has been pulled in place. The conjunctiva may be reattached with either fibrin glue or 8-0 vicryl with buried knots. We prefer fibrin glue for being faster and having a better cosmesis (Fig. 8.10).

Fig. 8.10 Conjuctival limbal scar after closure with fibrin glue on first postoperative day

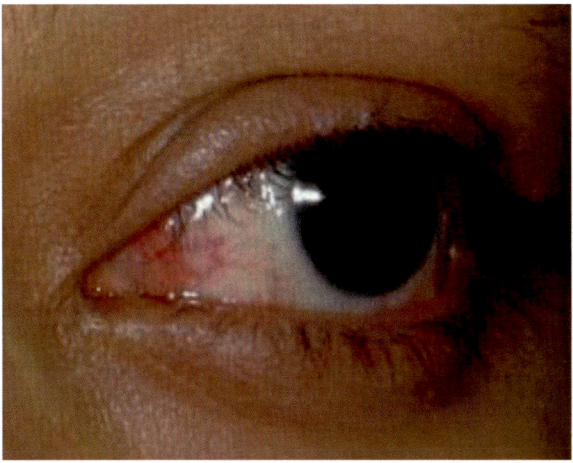

Conjunctival closure should be considered an important step as poorly apposed conjunctiva can give rise to an unsightly scar. Bunching of conjunctiva should be avoided, and Tenon's capsule should not be included in the suture while closing conjunctiva. If excessive manipulation has occurred, the Tenon's capsule may be closed in a separate layer below the conjunctiva. If conjunctiva is tight due to a long-standing deviation or scarring, it may be recessed to prevent reduction of the effect of muscle recession.

8.6   Postoperative Management

A tight bandage after surgery may reduce incidence of postoperative edema. The patient is prescribed an oral analgesic and anti-inflammatory medication for 3–5 days. Topical antibiotic, surface-acting steroid (like fluorometholone or lotepre-dnol), and lubricants are prescribed for 3–4 weeks. Post-op discomfort and foreign body sensation are common and transient. They may however persist with exposed sutures, prolapsed Tenon's capsule, or poor conjunctival closure. They have been addressed in Chap. 10.

8.7   Summary

- Strabismus surgery on horizontal recti is simple and gratifying which can be successfully executed even in a modest operating theater.
- It is advisable to have an anesthetist standby while performing surgery under local anesthesia due to possibility of oculocardiac reflex.
- The surgeon should confirm the informed consent, patient identity, and surgical plan himself before proceeding with surgery.
- Recession and resection are the most commonly performed surgeries.

- A good conjunctival incision provides adequate exposure without compromising cosmesis.
- Dissecting under direct visualization, avoiding injury to muscle sheath, engaging the entire muscle without leaving residual fibers, and freeing the muscle from surrounding attachments are some of the steps to enhance surgical results.
- Properly securing full thickness of the muscle with sutures at both borders, before detaching it, would prevent muscle loss and slippage.
- Hang-back, hemi-hang-back, and adjustable suture techniques are modifications of conventional recession useful for achieving more precise surgical outcomes.

8.8   Multiple Choice Questions

1. A 30-year-old man with 1-year-old partially recovered sixth nerve paresis of right side has RET and diplopia *only* in dextroversion. His diplopia and deviation are constant for 6 months. There is mild limitation of abduction of RE, and forced duction testing reveals no restriction. Most appropriate management option is
   (a) RMR rec + RLR res
   (b) LMR rec
   (c) Transposition of RSR and RIR to RLR insertion
   (d) Faden on LMR

Answer: (d) This patient has diplopia only in dextroversion and hence requires gaze selective surgery, i.e., Faden (retroequatorial myopexy) of the yoke (synergist in other eye) muscle. Yoke of the paralyzed RLR is LMR. Options "a" and "b" may correct the deviation but would also induce a deviation in primary gaze which is currently unaffected. Option "c" is indicated in complete palsy where the action of paralyzed muscle is negligible.

2. Which of the following is a strengthening procedure
   (a) Marginal myotomy
   (b) Tenotomy
   (c) Advancement
   (d) Recession

Answer: (c) Advancement is strengthening procedure which may be done with or without resection. All other options are weakening procedures.

3. Adjustable sutures are recommended for strabismus surgery in all of the following conditions EXCEPT
   (a) Thyroid eye disease
   (b) Post trauma surgery
   (c) Repeat surgery
   (d) Sensory exotropia

Answer: (d) Adjustable sutures are recommended whenever surgical results are unpredictable like in the first three options. In sensory exotropia, usually the neuromuscular components are intact, and surgical result is predictable. An overcorrection is planned, and slight variation in outcome does not warrant an additional procedure.

4. Which incision is best suited for beginners and occasional strabismus surgeons
   (a) Limbal incision with radial extensions
   (b) Fornix incision
   (c) Over the muscle incision
   (d) Paralimbal incision between the limbus and insertion

Answer: (a) The limbal incision provides good exposure, requires minimal assistance, and does not disturb the relationship between the conjunctiva and Tenon's capsule as both are firmly adherent at limbus. This incision is also suited for additional modifications like adjustable sutures, displacements, and transpositions.

5. Forced duction test (FDT) is performed to identify the presence of restrictive component in strabismus. Which of the following statement is true about it?
   (a) It is best performed under general anesthesia.
   (b) The patient is asked to look toward the direction of action of muscle being tested, e.g., adduction for medial rectus.
   (c) If full range of movement is not possible, the test is negative.
   (d) If full range of movement is possible, the cause of limited motility is probably paralytic.

Answer: (d) FDT can be performed as an office procedure after topical anesthesia, in fact muscle relaxants given during general anesthesia may cause the test to become falsely negative. The patient is asked to look in the direction of suspected limited duction, i.e., if medial rectus fibrosis is suspected, the patient would be instructed to abduct the eye to the maximum. If full range of movement is not possible, the test is positive, and the cause is restrictive. If full range is possible, the test is negative and the cause is paralytic.

References

1. Modarres M, Parvaresh MM, Hashemi M, Peyman GA. Inadvertent globe perforation during retrobulbar injection in high myopes. Int Ophthalmol. 1997;21:179–85.
2. Duker JS, Belmont JB, Benson WE, Brooks HL Jr, Brown GC, Federman JL, Fischer DH, Tasman WS. Inadvertent globe perforation during retrobulbar and peribulbar anesthesia. Patient characteristics, surgical management, and visual outcome. Ophthalmology. 1991;98(4):519–26.
3. Tejedor J, Ogallar C, Rodríguez JM. Surgery for esotropia under topical anesthesia. Ophthalmology. 2010;117(10):1883–8.
4. Dahlmann-Noor AH, Cosgrave E, Lowe S, Bailly M, Vivian AJ. Brimonidine and apraclonidine as vasoconstrictors in adjustable strabismus surgery. J AAPOS. 2009;13(2):123–6.

5. Mojon DS. Comparison of a new, minimally invasive strabismus surgery technique with the usual limbal approach for rectus muscle recession and plication. Br J Ophthalmol. 2007;91(1):76–82.

6. von Noorden GK, Campos EC. Principles of surgical treatment. In: von Noorden GK, Campos EC, editors. Binocular vision and ocular motility. 6th ed. St. Louis: Mosby; 2002. p. 566–631.

7. Agrawal S, Singh V, Gupta SK, Agrawal S. Comparison between limbal (von Noorden) and para limbal (Santiago) conjunctival incisions for adjustable recessions of horizontal recti. Nepal J Ophthalmol. 2013;5(2):220–5.

8. von Noorden GK. Modification of the limbal approach to surgery of the rectus muscles. Arch Ophthalmol. 1969;82:349–50.

9. Santiago AP, Isenberg SJ, Neumann D. The paralimbal approach with deferred conjunctival closure for adjustable strabismus surgery. Ophthalmic Surg Lasers. 1998;29:151–6.

10. Swan KC, Talbot T. Recession under Tenon's capsule. Arch Ophthalmol. 1954;51:32–45.

11. Parks MM. Fornix incision for horizontal rectus muscle surgery. Am J Ophthalmol. 1968;65(6):907–15.

12. Clark RA, Rosenbaum AL. Instrument induced measurement errors during strabismus surgery. J AAPOS. 1999;3(1):18–25.

13. Agrawal S, Singh V, Yadav A, Bangwal S, Katiyar V. Modified adjustable suture hang-back recession: description of technique and comparison with conventional adjustable hang-back recession. Indian J Ophthalmol. 2017;65:1183–6.

14. Lueder GT, Scott WE, Kutschke PJ, Keech RV. Long-term results of adjustable suture surgery for strabismus secondary to thyroid ophthalmopathy. Ophthalmology. 1992;99:993–7.

15. Park YC, Chun BY, Kwon JY. Comparison of the stability of postoperative alignment in sensory exotropia: adjustable versus non-adjustable surgery. Korean J Ophthalmol. 2009;23:277–80.

16. Bishop F, Doran RM. Adjustable and non-adjustable strabismus surgery: a retrospective case-matched study. Strabismus. 2004;12:3–11.

17. Agrawal S, Singh V, Singh P. Adjustable recessions in horizontal comitant strabismus: a pilot study. Indian J Ophthalmol. 2015;63:611–3.

18. Tripathi A, Haslett R, Marsh IB. Strabismus surgery: adjustable sutures—good for all? Eye. 2003;17:739–42.

19. Flynn JT. The adjustable suture: a clinician's experience. Pediatric ophthalmology and strabismus: transactions of the New Orleans Academy of Ophthalmology. New York: Raven Press; 1986. p. 245–6.

20. Keech VR. Adjustable suture strabismus surgery. In: Duane TD, Jaeger EA, editors. Duane's clinical ophthalmology, vol. 6. Philadelphia, PA: Lippincott Williams and Wilkins; 2009.

21. Bleik JH, Karam VY. Comparison of the immediate with the 24-hour postoperative prism and cover measurements in adjustable muscle surgery: is immediate postoperative adjustment reliable? J AAPOS. 2004;8(6):528–33.

22. Velez FG, Chan TK, Vives T, Chou T, Clark RA, Keyes M, et al. Timing of postoperative adjustment in adjustable suture strabismus surgery. J AAPOS. 2001;5(3):178–83.

23. Morris RJ, Luff AJ. Adjustable sutures in squint surgery. Br J Ophthalmol. 1992;76:560–2.

24. MacEwan CJ, Lee JP, Fells P. Aetiology and management of the 'detached' rectus muscle. Br J Ophthalmol. 1992;76:131–6.

Botulinum Toxin in Strabismus

9

Carol P. S. Lam, Joyce Chan, Winnie W. Y. Lau,
and Jason C. S. Yam

9.1   Introduction

Temporary chemodenervation using botulinum toxin injection is a useful option in management of strabismus patients with good binocularity in whom the deviation is expected to naturally recover. Ease of procedure, minimal complications, and reversibility make it a promising management option.

9.2   About the Toxin

Botulinum toxin (BoNT) is a potent neurotoxin that is produced by bacterium, *Clostridium botulinum*. Of the different antigenic botulinum toxins produced by different strains of this bacteria, only types A and B have been developed for commercial use in routine clinical practice, of which type A is used in ophthalmology. It is produced by various companies and the dried toxin requires reconstitution with saline. The packaging, safety margins, potency, and dosages of different preparations may vary [1–3]. The dosages mentioned in the chapter are of BOTOX®, (onabotulinum toxin A, Allergan, Inc., Irvine, CA) the most widely available product (Fig. 9.1).

C. P. S. Lam · J. Chan · W. W. Y. Lau
Hong Kong Eye Hospital, Kowloon, Hong Kong

J. C. S. Yam (✉)
Hong Kong Eye Hospital, Kowloon, Hong Kong

Department of Ophthalmology and Visual Sciences, The Chinese University of Hong Kong, Shatin, Hong Kong
e-mail: yamcheuksing@cuhk.edu.hk

© Springer Nature Singapore Pte Ltd. 2019
S. Agrawal (ed.), *Strabismus*, https://doi.org/10.1007/978-981-13-1126-0_9

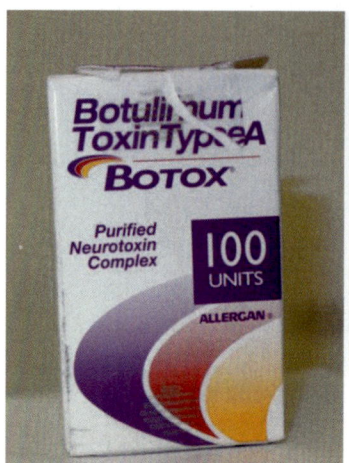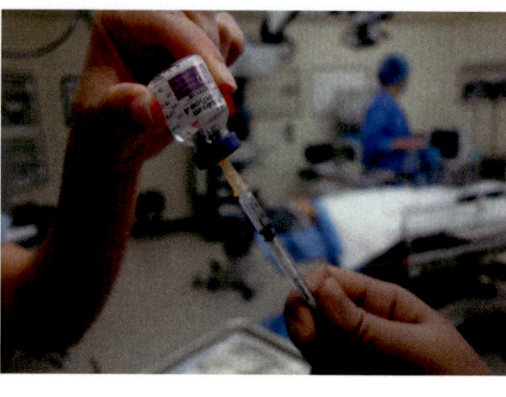

Fig. 9.1 Botulinum toxin A

9.2.1 Mechanism of Action

BoNT-A interferes with the release of acetylcholine into the neuromuscular junction and thus prevents muscle contraction [4]. Its use for strabismus was described in 1980s, and a single shot of BoNT-A can cause muscle paralysis lasting for weeks to months [5]. Its duration depends on various factors, including the nature of disease, method, and the dosage of the medication. The effect starts within 3–4 days and maximum effect is seen at about 7 days after injection. Once the toxin is effective, there may be an initial period of overcorrection depending on the strength of the antagonist.

With overcorrection there occurs contraction of the antagonist with stretching of the paralyzed muscle. Meanwhile, the length of the paralyzed muscle and its antagonist changes, and the length-tension curves within these muscles also change. A change in sarcomere density is also seen on histology. As the effect of BoNT-A wears off, few of these changes persist, and a resultant change to the ocular alignment occurs ("the after-effect") [6]. The long-term correction of strabismus may be thus be attributed to (a) temporary motor alignment causing sufficient strengthening of sensory fusion to overcome the motor instability, (b) recovery of motor instability occurring over a period of time, (c) overcoming of early contractures by induced paralysis, and (d) the permanent changes in muscle.

9.3 Indications

BoNT-A may be used when (a) assessment of deviation is unreliable, (b) surgical outcome is unpredictable, (c) palsy is recovering, or (d) deviation is small. Common indications of botulinum toxin in strabismus are listed in the Text Box 9.1 [7].

Text Box 9.1: Indications of Botulinum Toxin
1. Concomitant deviations
   (a) Infantile ET
   (b) Intermittent XT
   (c) Associated neurological conditions (like cerebral palsy)
   (d) Retreatment/augmentation of surgical effect
2. Incomitant deviations
   (a) Sixth nerve palsy
   (b) Fourth nerve palsy.
   (c) Thyroid ophthalmopathy (restrictive squint)
3. Nystagmus

9.3.1 Concomitant Deviation

9.3.1.1 Infantile Esotropia

Bimedial injection of botulinum toxin before 12 months of age is reported to be useful in patients with infantile esotropia with demonstrable stereopsis when the child is older [8]. Although the overall success rate by injections is much lower compared to surgery, botulinum has the advantage of avoiding overcorrection and delaying surgery till a time accurate measurements can be made [9]. The dosage is 2.5 units in each medial rectus (MR).

9.3.1.2 Intermittent Exotropia

Botulinum toxin has shown promising results in childhood intermittent exotropia [10, 11]. Adults with initial small deviation have a better response than those with larger deviation [12]. The initial dosage is 2.5 units in each lateral rectus (LR).

9.3.1.3 Cerebral Palsy

The deviation in conditions like cerebral palsy is often variable and unpredictable. They are at high risk for general anesthesia, and surgical outcomes are suboptimal. We and many others like to maintain ocular alignment in these patients with repeated botulinum injections till their systemic condition becomes stable [13]. Lesser dose should be given initially ranging from 1.5 units in each MR (for ET) to 2–2.5 units in each LR (for XT).

9.3.1.4 Retreatment and Augmentation Surgery

The toxin is a useful adjunct to management of residual or consecutive deviations with many studies showing similar outcome to resurgery [14–16]. Injecting the toxin into the recessed horizontal rectus muscle further weakens the muscle for supra maximal effect [17]. Where multiple muscle surgery is being considered, using botulinum instead of recession helps preserve its anterior ciliary artery thus preventing anterior segment ischemia.

9.3.2 Incomitant Deviation

9.3.2.1 Sixth Nerve Palsy

Botulinum prevents diplopia and contractures of medial rectus during the recovery of sixth nerve paralysis but has no effect on the eventual outcome [18, 19]. Quality of life of the patient improves with enlargement of the diplopia-free field and better cosmesis [18, 20]. It is also believed to reduce the length of morbidity [20, 21]. In permanent palsy the role of botulinum is limited, and surgery should be considered.

9.3.2.2 Fourth Nerve Palsy

Botulinum injection is less commonly used in superior oblique palsy than in sixth nerve palsy as the results are often less predictable. The yoke muscle (inferior rectus of the other eye) may be injected [22].

9.3.2.3 Thyroid Ophthalmopathy (Restrictive Strabismus)

The inferior rectus and medial rectus are most commonly enlarged, causing restrictive strabismus and intolerable diplopia. Botulinum toxin allows patients to maintain binocular single vision during the acute part of the disease until their ophthalmopathy stabilizes enabling strabismus surgery. Botulinum is given in the inferior or medial rectus or both depending on the deviation in acute phase. Surgery may be avoided in a few patients [23]. An additional benefit is decrease in the intraocular pressure due to the improvement in ocular deviation [24].

9.3.3 Nystagmus

Acquired nystagmus is often associated with impaired visual function, due to the excessive movement of retinal images. Failure of the visual cortex to adapt to nystagmus results in oscillopsia, which may be incapacitating. The treatment was initially described as a retrobulbar botulinum toxin injection, but it is safer to inject one or more horizontal muscles directly (for horizontal nystagmus) for an effect lasting 3–4 months [25–27].

9.4   Injection Technique

The most common technique of BoNT-A injection into extra ocular muscles is under EMG (electromyograph) guidance through a topically anesthetized conjunctiva [6] (Fig. 9.2). A specially designed 27 G needle (with the shaft coated and connected to the electrode) is introduced through the conjunctiva, parallel to the surface of the sclera in order to avoid penetration into the globe (Fig. 9.3). The patient is first asked to look in the opposite direction to the action of the muscle being injected. When the needle is in the muscle belly, the patient is then asked to look in the direction of action of the extraocular muscle being injected. Meanwhile, there will be an increase in the signal output from the EMG, confirming the correct location of the needle. Slow injection of BoNT-A is then made [6].

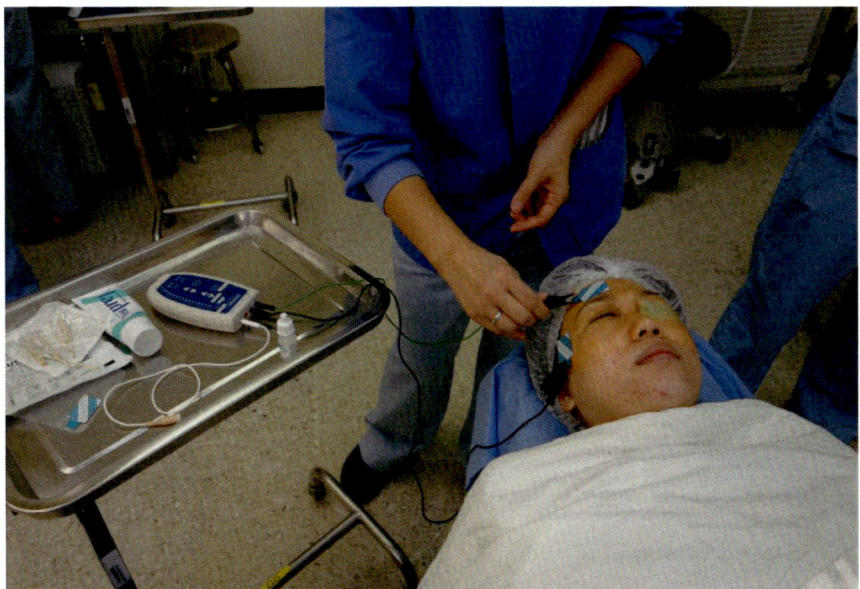

Fig. 9.2 EMG-guided botox injection

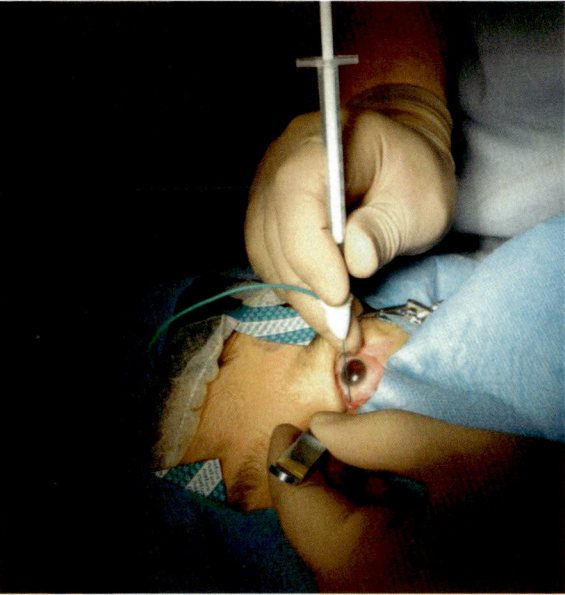

Fig. 9.3 A specially designed 27 G needle is introduced through the conjunctiva, parallel to the surface of the sclera in order to avoid penetration into the globe

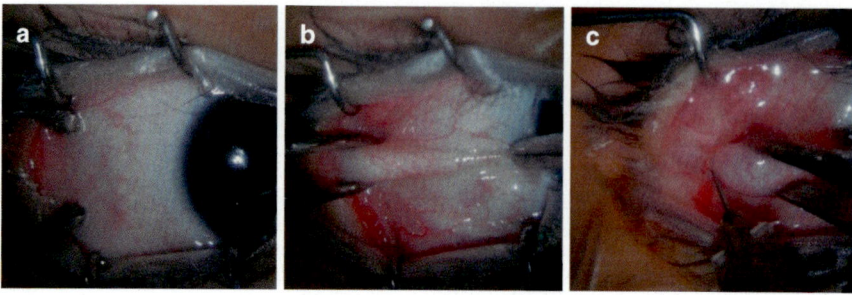

Fig. 9.4 Transconjunctival injection of botulinum. (**a**) For injection into the lateral rectus muscle, the patient asked to adduct the eye after instillation of topical anesthesia. (**b**) The globe is further adducted if required by holding it at the limbus and the lateral rectus grasped transconjunctivally with the fixation forcep about 10 mm from the limbus. (**c**) The muscle is slightly pulled up and the botulinum injection given after advancing the needle by about 3–5 mm at the posterior limit of bunched up muscle

Several other techniques for injection have been described (see Text Box 9.2) [28–32]. Some authors of this book give the injection transconjunctivally with satisfactory results after grasping the muscle with Graefe fixation forceps, which is less traumatic compared to the conventionally used Mendonca forceps [29] (Fig. 9.4).

Text Box 9.2: Different Techniques of Botulinum Toxin Injection
- EMG guided through a topically anesthetized conjunctiva [5]
- Transconjunctivally without EMG and without holding the muscle [31, 32]
- Under direct vision into a muscle during squint surgery
- Under direct vision through a conjunctival incision prepared for the BoNT-A injection [30]
- Sub-Tenon's with lacrimal cannula alongside a muscle [28]
- Transconjunctivally after grasping the muscle with forceps and bunching it up [29]

9.5   Complications and Contraindications

Common complications like ptosis and induced vertical deviation occur due to spread of the toxin to other extra ocular muscles or levator palpebral superioris. Other complications like subconjunctival hemorrhage, muscle hematoma, retrobulbar hemorrhage, and globe perforation are rare and caused by inappropriate injection technique. Among all, ptosis was the most commonly documented complication, the occurrence rate ranged from 8.4% to 53% of cases. It is found to have higher frequency in children than in adults due to the small orbits and higher doses of toxin used [33]. There is one case report each of bullous retinal detachment and vitreous hemorrhage with inadvertent intraocular injection of botulinum toxin A [34, 35]. Theoretical systemic risks of botulinum toxin include diffuse muscle weakness, dysphonia, dysarthria, dysphagia, urinary incontinence, and dyspnea. These have never been reported with the ocular use of botulinum toxin; however, a history of myasthenia gravis must be ruled out.

There are no reported contraindications for the use BoNT. The only contraindication may be a known allergy to the toxin.

9.6   Summary

- Botulinum toxin (BoNT) is a neurotoxin produced by bacteria *Clostridium botulinum*. BoNT acts by preventing presynaptic release of acetylcholine at neuromuscular junction. BoNT type A is most commonly used in ophthalmology for temporary chemodenervation.
- Common indications for use of BoNT-A include infantile esotropia, strabismus with cerebral palsy, abducens nerve palsy, thyroid ophthalmopathy, and nystagmus.
- Ptosis and iatrogenic vertical deviations are common side effects of BoNT-A injections.
- Ease of procedure, minimal complications, and reversibility make BoNT-A injection a viable alternative to surgery in selected cases.

9.7   Case Discussion

Case 1. The entire spectrum of botulinum injection usage is depicted by this patient of infantile esotropia. The initial photograph is of the child at the age of 2.5 years with a 40 PD ET. Child was alternating and was uncooperative for binocular function assessment. Parents being unwilling for surgery, he received 2.5 units of botulinum toxin in both medial recti. The deviation was corrected, but the child developed right upper lid ptosis at 1 week. The ptosis gradually recovered and the ocular alignment was maintained for up to 9 months post injection when the child started redeveloping alternating ET. At this time his stereo acuity was 100 s on Randot. The temporary alignment provided enough stimulus for binocular functions to develop. The child eventually underwent strabismus surgery (medial rectus recession both eyes) at 3.5 years of age. The child is straight at the age of 5 years with a stereo acuity of 40 s.

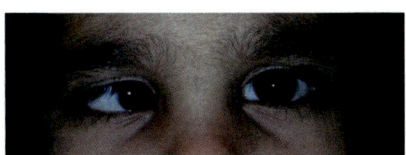

Preinjection

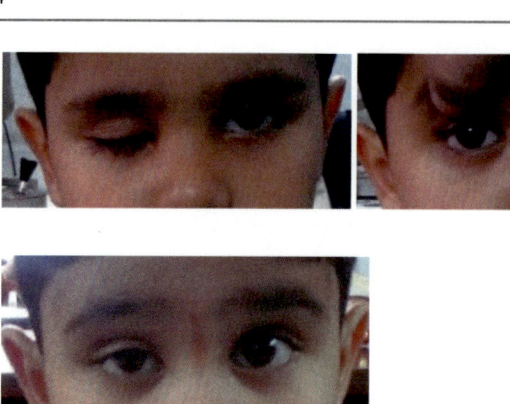

7 days post injection

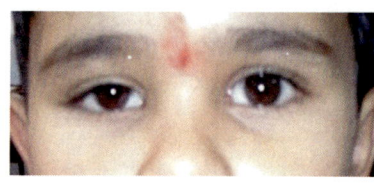

4 weeks post injection

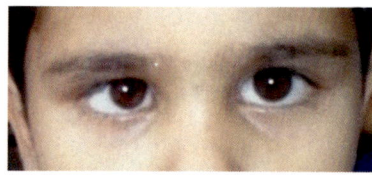

5 months post injection

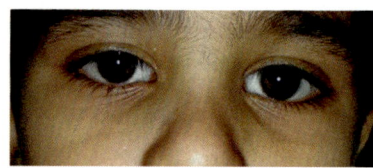

12 months post injection

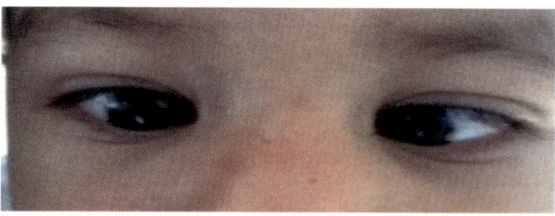

12 months after surgery

Case 2. This child underwent 2.5 units botulinum toxin injection in both medial recti at the age of 1 year for infantile esotropia. The child became orthotropic at 1 week post injection and has remained so for 4 years now. His stereopsis for near at 5 years of age is 60 s.

Preinjection

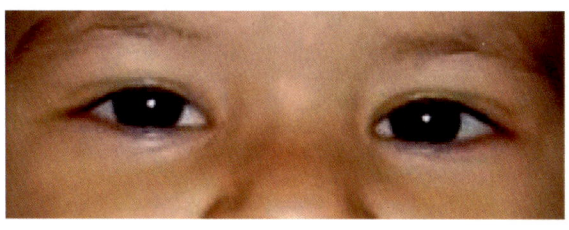
4 years post injection.

9.8   Multiple Choice Questions

1. Which of the following statements is true with regard to use of botulinum toxin in ophthalmology?
   (a) Single injection provides long-term control of nystagmus in children.
   (b) It should be offered as first choice of treatment in a healthy 4-year-old with infantile esotropia.
   (c) It should be considered in children with unstable deviations associated with neurological conditions or those unfit or unwilling for surgery.
   (d) It should not be considered in patients with paralytic deviations for fear of increasing diplopia.

Answer: (c) Repeated injections are required in nystagmus. Definite management of infantile esotropia is surgical. Botulinum should be used in children with unstable deviations, cerebral palsy, and in those unfit or unwilling for surgery. It is useful in paralytic deviations and the direct antagonist or the yoke of the paralyzed muscle is injected to control diplopia.

2. Regarding the dosage and preparation of botulinum toxin, which of the following statements are true?
   (a) Once prepared the vial may be used up to 2 weeks.
   (b) The toxin should be vigorously agitated after the diluent is added to ensure homogenous solution.
   (c) The usual dosage of Botox is about 2.5 units per muscle; however, it varies according to the preparation and indication.
   (d) It is unusual for ptosis to occur after injection.

Answer: (c) Only freshly prepared toxin should be used within 4 h of preparation. The toxin is sensitive to agitation and should be mixed gently. The dosage varies in different preparations and indications. Ptosis is the commonest complication to occur post injection.

References

1. Wheeler A, Smith HS. Botulinum toxins: mechanisms of action, antinociception and clinical applications. Toxicology. 2013;306:124–46.
2. Aoki KR. A comparison of the safety margins of botulinum neurotoxin serotype A, B and F in mice. Toxicon. 2001;39:1815–20.

3. Brin MF, James C, Maltman J. Botulinum toxin type A products are not interchangeable: a review of the evidence. Biologics. 2014;8:227–41.
4. Levy NS, Lowenthal DT. Application of botulinum toxin to clinical therapy: advances and cautions. Am J Ther. 2012;19:281–96.
5. Scott AB. Botulinum toxin injection into extraocular muscles as an alternative to strabismus surgery. Ophthalmology. 1980;87(10):1044–9.
6. Kowal L, Wong E, Yahalom C. Botulinum toxin in the treatment of strabismus. A review of its use and effects. Disabil Rehabil. 2007;29(23):1823–31.
7. Rowe FJ, Noonan CP. Botulinum toxin for the treatment of strabismus. Cochrane Database Syst Rev. 2012;15(2):CD006499.
8. McNeer KW, Tucker MG, Guerry CH, Spencer RF. Incidence of stereopsis after treatment of infantile esotropia with botulinum toxin A. J Pediatr Ophthalmol Strabismus. 2003;40:288–92.
9. de Alba Campomanes AG, Binenbaum G, Campomanes Eguiarte G. Comparison of botulinum toxin with surgery as primary treatment for infantile esotropia. J AAPOS. 2010;14(2):111–6.
10. Spencer RF, et al. Botulinum toxin management of childhood intermittent exotropia. Ophthalmology. 1997;104(11):1762–7.
11. Etezad Razavi M, Sharifi M, Armanfar F. Efficacy of botulonim toxin in the treatment of intermittent exotropia. Strabismus. 2014;22(4):176–81.
12. Carruthers JD, Kennedy RA, Bagaric D. Botulinum versus adjustable suture surgery in the treatment of horizontal misalignment in adult patients lacking fusion. Arch Ophthalmol. 1990;108(10):1432–5.
13. Cronemberger MF, Mendonça TS, Bicas HE. Botulinum toxin treatment for horizontal strabismus in children with cerebral palsy. Arq Bras Oftalmol. 2006;69(4):523–9.
14. Tejedor J, Rodriguez JM. Early retreatment of infantile esotropia: comparison of reoperation and botulinum toxin. Br J Ophthalmol. 1999;83:783–7.
15. Tejedor J, Rodriguez JM. Retreatment of children after surgery for acquired esotropia: reoperation versus botulinum injection. Br J Ophthalmol. 1998;82:110–4.
16. Dawson ELM, Marshman WE, Lee JP. Role of botulinum toxin A in surgically overcorrected exotropia. J AAPOS. 1999;3:269–71.
17. Ozkan SB, Topaloğlu A, Aydin S. The role of botulinum toxin A in augmentation to the effect of recession and/or resection surgery. J AAPOS. 2006;10(2):124–7.
18. Lee J, Harris S, Cohen J, Cooper K, MacEwen C, Jones S. Results of a prospective randomized trial of botulinum toxin therapy in acute unilateral sixth nerve palsy. J Pediatr Ophthalmol Strabismus. 1994;31(5):283–6.
19. Holmes JM, Beck RW, Kip KE, Droste PJ, Leske DA. Botulinum toxin treatment versus conservative management in acute traumatic sixth nerve palsy or paresis. J AAPOS. 2000;4(3):145–9.
20. Lee JP. Modern management of VI nerve palsy. Aust N Z J Ophthalmol. 1992;20:41.
21. Murray AD. Early botulinum toxin treatment of acute sixth nerve palsy. Eye. 1991;5:45.
22. Garnham L, Lawson JM, et al. Botulinum toxin in fourth nerve palsies. Aus N Z J Ophthalmol. 1997;25:31–5.
23. Lyons CJ, Vickers SF, Lee JP. Botulinum toxin therapy in dysthyroid strabismus. Eye. 1990;4:538–40.
24. Kikawa DO, Cruz RC, Christian WK, Rikkers S, Weinreb RN, Levi L, et al. A toxin injection for restrictive myopathy of thyroid related orbitopathy: effects in intraocular pressure. Am J Ophthalmol. 2003;135(4):427–31.
25. Helveston EM, Pogrebniak AE. Treatment of acquired nystagmus with botulinum A toxin. Am J Ophthalmol. 1988;106:9–16.
26. Hobson F, Rowe F. Management of nystagmus by surgery and botulinum toxin options: a review. Br Ir Orthopt J. 2009;6:28–33.
27. Lennerstrand G, Nordbø OA, Tian S, Eriksson-Derouet B, Ali T. Treatment of strabismus and nystagmus with botulinum toxin type A. An evaluation of effects and complications. Acta Ophthalmol Scand. 1998;76(1):27.

28. Ly K, Chao AN. Subtenon injection of botulinum toxin for treatment of traumatic sixth nerve palsy. J Pediatr Ophthalmol Strabismus. 2003;40(1):27–30.
29. Mendonca TF, Cronemberger MF, Lopes MC, Nakanami CR, Bicas HE. Electromyography assistance and Mendoca's forceps—a comparison between two methods of botulinum toxin A injection into the extraocular muscle. Arq Bras Oftalmol. 2005;68(2):245–9.
30. Campos EC. Pharmacological treatment of strabismus. In: Lennerstrand G, Ygge J, editors. Advances in strabismus research: basic and clinical aspects, Wenner Gren international series, vol. 78. London: Portland Press; 2000. p. 167.
31. Sanjari MS, Falavarjani KG, Kashkouli MB, Aghai GH, Nojomi M, Rostami H. Botulinum toxin injection with and without electromyographic assistance for treatment of abducens nerve palsy: a pilot study. J Pediatr Ophthalmol Strabismus. 2008;12(3):259–62.
32. Benabent EC, Garcia Hermosa P, Arrazola MT, Alio y Sanz JL. Botulinum toxin injection without electromyographic assistance. J Pediatr Ophthalmol Strabismus. 2002;39:231–4.
33. Rowe F, Noonan C. Complications of Botulinum toxin A and their adverse effects. Strabismus. 2009;17(4):139–42.
34. Liu M, Lee HC. Retinal detachment from inadvertent intraocular injection of botulinum toxin A. Am J Ophthalmol. 2004;137(1):201–2.
35. Agrawal S, Singh V, Gupta SK, Vinod Kumar BM. Vitreous haemorrhage following inadvertent intraocular injection of botulinum toxin. Oman J Ophthalmol. 2015;8:79–80.

Complications of Strabismus Surgery

10

Swati Phuljhele, Rohit Saxena, Pradeep Sharma, and Manu Saini

10.1 Introduction

Over the years, the strabismus surgery has undergone improvement in terms of both efficacy and safety. Although serious complications are fortunately rare, no surgery is devoid of risk. It is important for surgeons to be aware of the incidence of complications and various factors that may increase the risk. The complications range from preoperative glitches like wrong surgery to postoperative complications like undesired correction and infection.

10.2 Preoperative Complication

10.2.1 Error in Patient Identity or Surgical Plan

Even though it may appear unrealistic, mistake in the identity of the patient is a possibility in a busy operation theatre. There can be no greater misfortune for the operating team than to perform surgery on the incorrect patient, eye or muscle. The patient particulars and the surgical plan must be reconfirmed by the surgeon himself immediately prior to starting the surgery. These errors are commoner when the surgeon moves between multiple operating rooms and the muscles to be operated have not been marked preoperatively [1]. It should be kept in mind that these errors are considered as negligence (and not complication) legally.

S. Phuljhele (✉) · R. Saxena · P. Sharma · M. Saini
Dr. Rajendra Prasad Centre for Ophthalmic Sciences, All India Institute of Medical Sciences (AIIMS), New Delhi, India

© Springer Nature Singapore Pte Ltd. 2019
S. Agrawal (ed.), *Strabismus*, https://doi.org/10.1007/978-981-13-1126-0_10

10.3   Per-Operative Complications

10.3.1 Identification of the Muscle

Sometimes if the surgical exposure is inadequate or due to globe rotation, an inexperienced surgeon may pick up a wrong muscle for surgery. The confusion occurs most commonly between the lateral rectus and inferior oblique. The best way to confirm the identity of the muscle is to give the muscle a gentle tug and observe the effect on the eye. It is advisable to increase the size of incision and identify the muscle under direct visualization. Placing fixation sutures (Chap. 8) also helps by providing an axis guide and preventing undue rotation of the globe which may happen during surgery.

10.3.2 Haemorrhage

Per-operative haemorrhage compromises surgical field visibility and increases the chances of postoperative scarring. Common cause of bleeding is disruption of the muscle sheath and injury to the muscle during dissection. Blind dissection in the area where the muscle insertion is expected should not be done (Chap. 8). Other causes of bleeding are inadvertent injury to vortex veins and scarring from previous surgery. Topical vasoconstrictors, bipolar cautery and careful dissection help decrease the incidence of bleeding [2].

Text Box 10.1: Causes of Lost and Slipped Muscle
- Passing sutures only through muscle sheath without including the muscle fibres
- Inadvertently cutting sutures while disinserting muscle
- Tearing of tight muscle due to extensive tension—Pulled-in-two syndrome (PITS)
- Superficial bites while passing sutures through sclera
- Risk factors like advanced age, restrictive strabismus, prior radiation or surgery

10.3.3 Lost/Slipped/Severed Muscle and PITS

A *lost muscle* is characterized by the absence of any attachment of the muscle tendon or its sheath to the sclera [3, 4]. The muscle along with its sheath recoils posteriorly through the Tenon's capsule. In *slipped muscle* the tendon retracts posteriorly within the muscle sheath. The sheath remains empty and attached to the sclera at the chosen insertion site [5]. Common causes of lost and slipped muscle are listed in the Text Box 10.1 [6–8].

Sometimes when the muscle is too tight or fibrosed, it may retract uncontrollably after tenotomy or inadvertent myotomy/myectomy during dissection resulting in a *severed* muscle. The muscle may also get torn at the muscle-tendon junction as a result of excessive tension or pull on the muscle. This is termed as *pulled-in-two syndrome (PITS)* [6]. The medial rectus is the commonest muscle to retract posteriorly and difficult to recover thereafter as it has minimal attachments with surrounding muscles and a shorter arc of contact [4, 9].

A slipped muscle when discovered intraoperatively is easier to retrieve and secured to the sclera with full-thickness bites through the muscle. One should avoid pulling the Tenon's capsule or rotating the globe on the opposite side to get more exposure as this would cause the muscle to retract further back. In fact, the globe should be compressed or retro placed and then the posterior Tenon's capsule should be gently opened. The dissection should be directed towards the orbital apex and muscle should be explored. Similarly, a severed muscle is managed by careful identification, dissection from surrounding tissues and resuturing to the desired site [3].

In cases of PITS, the posterior detached part of the muscle is explored as described above. If found it can be sutured to the anterior part of the muscle that remains attached to the sclera or can be directly sutured to the sclera in a recessed position [10, 11].

If the exploration and retrieval fail, a delayed transposition surgery may be required in order to achieve alignment and ocular motility.

> *Clinical Tip: Before passing sutures through the muscle, it must be ensured that the entire width of the muscle is in the muscle hook and both borders are well visualized.*

10.3.4 Globe Perforation

Scleral perforation is one of the most severe and potentially devastating complications of strabismus surgery. The perforation typically occurs while passing the sutures through the sclera during reattaching the muscle. In case the perforation has occurred, one can still go ahead with rest of the surgery provided there is no vitreous loss and excessive manipulation is not needed. However intraoperative or postoperative dilated fundus examination is mandatory to look for any retinal tear. Retinopexy either with cryo or laser may be required to prevent further complications.

Dilated pupil indirect ophthalmoscopy performed after strabismus surgery has reported incidence of scleral perforation between 0.4% and 1.8% [12]. Its risk factors are thin sclera, high myopia, inexperienced surgeons and re-surgeries.

10.3.5 Oculocardiac Reflex

Oculocardiac reflex is characterized by sinus bradycardia, ectopic beats or sinus arrest during manipulation of extraocular muscles, specially the medial rectus. Prompt diagnosis should be followed by immediate release of the muscle. If it persists, intravenous atropine (0.15 mg/kg) is given. In recalcitrant cases, retrobulbar lignocaine is recommended to block the afferent loop.

For this reason a monitor should always be connected and an anaesthetist be present while performing strabismus surgery, even under local anaesthesia.

10.4 Postoperative Complications

10.4.1 Ocular Surface Complications

10.4.1.1 Corneal Dellen
Corneal dellen formation occurs when the tear film regularity is disturbed due to conjunctival swelling or its unsatisfactory approximation at limbus. It is commoner after medial rectus re-surgery or transposition procedures and responds well to aggressive lubrication [13].

10.4.1.2 Inclusion Cyst
Edge-to-edge conjunctival closure not only enhances postoperative cosmetic outcome; it also reduces the incidence of inclusion cyst formation. Inclusion cyst is usually non-tender, translucent and arises from inadvertent burying of conjunctiva while approximating the edges (Fig. 10.4). The risk factors include younger age and muscle recession procedures [14].

Treatment is not always indicated; cysts those are small and asymptomatic may be observed. However, cysts that form early in the postoperative period may become infected, necessitating antibiotic therapy and surgical excision [15, 16].

10.4.1.3 Prolapsed Tenon's Capsule
Exposed or prolapsed Tenon's tissue caused by improper apposition of the conjunctival edges results in unsightly scar. It can be managed by surgical excision of the prolapsed tissue (Fig. 10.1). Meticulous surgical dissection and paying attention to approximation of Tenon's capsule during incision closure may reduce its occurrence.

10.4.2 Lost or Slipped Muscle

Lost or slipped muscle may also present in the early postoperative period. The clinical manifestations of a lost muscle are more severe and appear earlier than those of a slipped muscle. Along with gross motility limitation, there is protrusion of the globe as patient attempts to move the eye in the direction of action of the lost muscle. This is due to a relaxation of the antagonist and the lack of pull of the lost muscle [11]. Magnetic resonance imaging (MRI) is preferred for localization of the muscle and determining presence or absence of its attachments to the globe [17–19]. When the

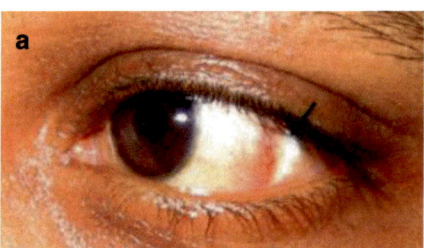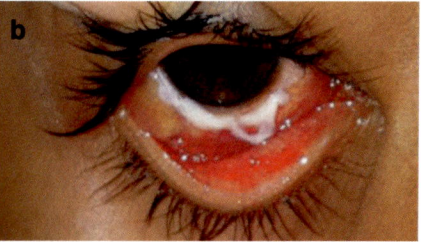

Fig. 10.1 (a) Wound gape and prolapsed Tenon's capsule (arrow) from fornix incision. (b) Prolapse of Tenon's capsule from limbal incision

diagnosis of slipped or lost muscle is suspected, surgical exploration is indicated. It has been recommended that the surgical exploration should not be delayed for more than 2 weeks to avoid contracture of the ipsilateral antagonist [17]. Tracing the path of the capsule posteriorly until the muscle body is found can usually retrieve the slipped muscle. To identify an empty muscle capsule in case of slipped muscle, a strabismus hook is passed under the attached tissue; if the muscle has slipped, a thin translucent sheath will allow the hook to be clearly visible. The empty capsule is followed posteriorly until the muscle fibres are found. The tendon fibres and overlying capsule are then secured with sutures to the desired site. The surgeon should also be prepared with a second plan in the form of transposition surgery, should the retrieval fail.

10.4.3 Overcorrection (Consecutive Strabismus)/Undercorrection (Residual Strabismus)

Unsatisfactory ocular alignment after surgery is a common postoperative complication. Inherent unpredictability of the procedure, incorrect preoperative evaluation or surgical dosage calculation, overlooking oblique muscle dysfunctions or other dynamic factors and improper surgical technique are frequent causes for early postoperative malalignment (Fig. 10.2). Each of these factors has been discussed in earlier chapters.

Unless the diagnosis of slipped or lost muscle is suspected, immediate corrective measures are not necessary. The patient needs to be reassured and re-evaluated later to determine if the outcome is unacceptable and requires re-surgery. Text Box 10.2 summarizes such unacceptable motor outcomes in common types of strabismus [20–22]. Botulinum toxin and prisms may be used in the interim in selected cases. Adjustable sutures enhance satisfactory outcomes as has been discussed in earlier chapters.

Text Box 10.2: Unacceptable Motor Outcomes [20–22]

Infantile ET	>20Δ ET or XT
XT	>15Δ ET
	Residual XT
Sensory strabismus	>10Δ XT
Incomitant strabismus	>10Δ deviation in primary or down gaze

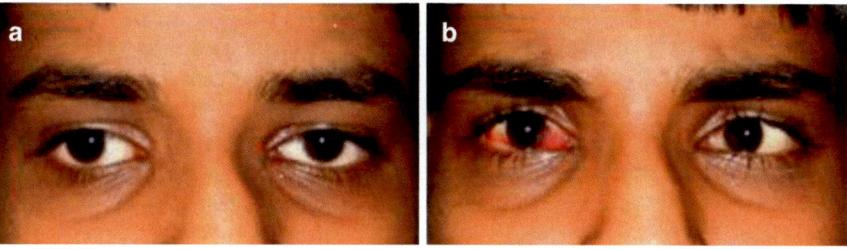

Fig. 10.2 (**a**) Fourteen-year-old boy with right eye exotropia, (**b**) following surgery (LR recession and MR resection) developed consecutive esotropia with diplopia

Late postoperative ocular malalignment of eyes that were aligned in the early postoperative period can usually be attributed to the type/cause of strabismus. Exodrift in X(T), reactivation of thyroid ophthalmopathy and progressive myopathy are few examples. Sometimes fibrosis of conjunctival scar may be a cause of late motility limitation.

10.4.4 Postoperative Diplopia

Early postoperative diplopia after strabismus surgery is distressing for the patient but is often not an unwelcome sign for the surgeon. In conditions like X(T), it may be acceptable, and in long-standing deviations, it may be a welcome sign with a potential of binocular recovery. Patient should be reassured and given time to fuse, suppress or ignore the second image. Frequently the patients are able to overcome the diplopia in a few days. Prisms should be considered only after few weeks.

Surgical realignment may be required after a few weeks if troublesome diplopia and deviation persist in primary and downgazes. Abnormal retinal correspondence may cause transient paradoxical diplopia in presence of orthotropia.

Surgeon should be aware of the possibility of postoperative diplopia in different types of strabismus like X(T), paralytic deviations, etc. and warn these patients prior to surgery. It is even better to make the patients experience diplopia by correcting or nearly correcting the deviation with prisms prior to surgery. This ensures that it does not come as a surprise and patients don't see it as a complication.

10.4.5 Change in Visual Acuity and Refractive Error

An observant patient may notice a change in visual acuity after strabismus surgery. This can be attributed to development of astigmatism due to alteration in corneal curvature as response to the reduction in tension of the recessed extraocular muscle transmitted via the sclera to the cornea [23, 24]. This phenomenon is commoner in restrictive strabismus and is usually transient [23, 25]. Change of glasses should be done only after 3 months of surgery [26].

10.4.6 Change in Palpebral Aperture

Horizontal muscle strabismus surgery is known to cause palpebral aperture (PA) changes [27, 28]. Recession of a horizontal rectus muscle causes widening of the PA while resection decreases its height. The amount change in PA may be related to the amount surgery done on rectus muscle (Fig. 10.3). Changes in PA also occur after surgery on vertical recti if attachments between the muscles and lid retractors are not severed [29]. Recession of vertical recti may cause widening of the aperture while resection may cause its narrowing.

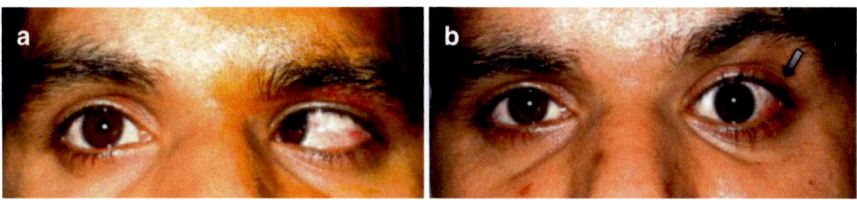

Fig. 10.3 (**a**) Case of left lateral rectus palsy underwent MR recession with half width transposition of vertical recti to LR, (**b**) postoperative satisfactory alignment in primary position with widening palpebral aperture

10.4.7 Retinal Detachment

Intraoperative scleral perforation during muscle reattachment may cause postoperative retinal detachment depending of the depth of the needle pass. All suspected perforations should be managed as discussed above in globe perforation. The incidence of detachment is reported to be 1.9% in presence of retinal tear [30].

10.4.8 Anterior Segment Ischaemia

The risk of anterior segment ischaemia is influenced by both patient susceptibility and the extent of the strabismus surgery. The most important patient risk factor is older age [31]. Other reported risk factors include atherosclerosis, blood dyscrasias, hyperviscosity syndromes, carotid artery ligation and Graves ophthalmopathy [32].

Anterior segment ischaemia may occur after transposition procedures, surgeries involving more than two recti simultaneously and vertical recti surgery on patients who have previously undergone horizontal surgery [33].

Vessel sparing surgery may prevent anterior segment ischaemia, but does not eliminate the risk entirely [34]. Muscle plication, an alternative to resection, has also been utilized in an effort to preserve ciliary vasculature.

Clinical features include severe ocular pain, corneal oedema, anterior segment flare and hypotony. It is managed by short course of systemic steroids and intensive application of topical steroids. Most patients recover iris circulation by 12 weeks with increased blood flow through the long posterior ciliary arteries.

10.4.9 Postoperative Infections

10.4.9.1 Suture Abscess and Granuloma

Suture abscess is usually seen within a week of surgery and is caused by contaminated suture. It presents as yellowish nodule with swelling and erythema over the suture site [35]. It usually needs to be drained followed by topical antibiotics. Granulomas on the other hand occur between 2 and 4 weeks of surgery due to foreign body reaction to suture material, cotton fibres, glove powder or a buried eye

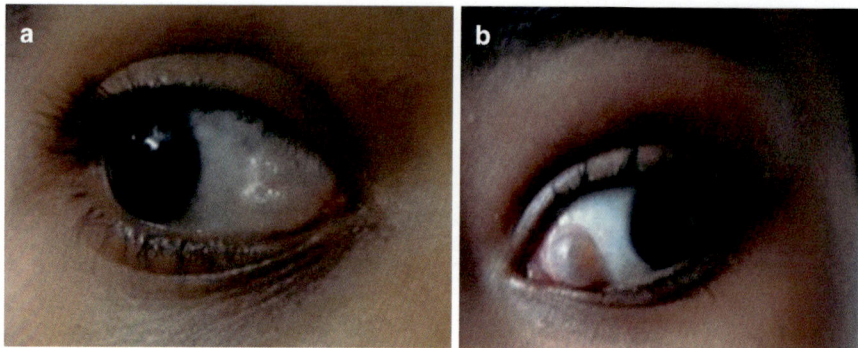

Fig. 10.4 Suture-related complications (**a**) Inclusion cyst (**b**) Suture granuloma

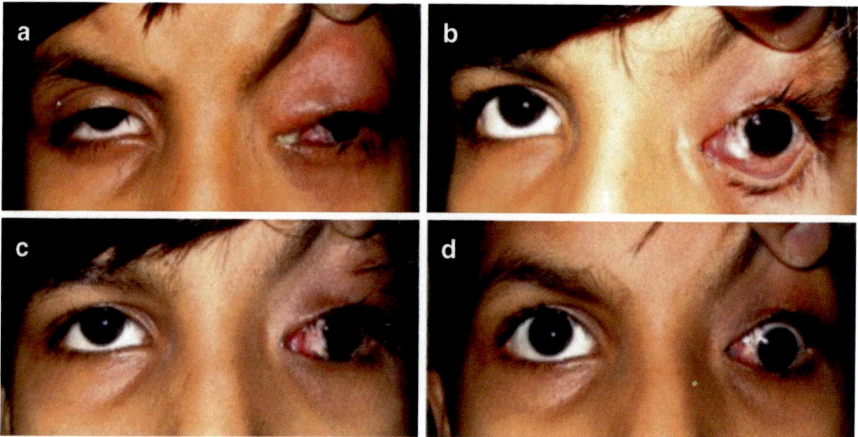

Fig. 10.5 Twelve-year old developed orbital cellulitis (**a, b**) after strabismus surgery for complete third nerve palsy which responded to systemic antibiotics (**c, d**)

lash [35] (Fig. 10.4). Majority of granulomas resolve with topical corticosteroids and surgical excision is seldom needed.

10.4.9.2 Orbital Cellulites and Endophthalmitis

Orbital cellulitis and endophthalmitis are rare but unfortunate complications of strabismus surgery (Fig. 10.5). Endophthalmitis is more common in presence of scleral perforation. Treatment involves aggressive topical, intravitreal and systemic antibiotics; vitrectomy may be required for nonresponsive endophthalmitis. CT scan is indicated in orbital cellulitis to identify any abscess which may need drainage [35].

10.5 Summary

- With evolution in surgical technique and instrumentation, the complications related to strabismus surgery have declined over time.
- Error in identification of extraocular muscle and per-operative haemorrhage following injury to muscle sheath are common with beginners.
- Muscle loss or slippage may occur per-operatively or in early postoperative period. Medial rectus muscle is more prone due to straighter orbital course and minimal surrounding attachments.
- Globe perforation, retinal detachment and anterior segment ischaemia are rare but sight threatening.
- Under- and overcorrections are common. Inherent unpredictability of the procedure, incorrect surgical planning or its execution are common causes of unexpected surgical outcome.

10.6 Multiple Choice Questions

1. Which of the following statement is *incorrect* regarding preoperative evaluation for strabismus surgery?
   (a) Prism adaptation test is avoidable in patients with no demonstrable binocularity.
   (b) Prism testing and evaluation of sensory status are useful to determine postoperative fusion ability and presence of ARC.
   (c) Assessment of deviation is incomplete without measuring associated features like presence of any A-V patterns, presence of accommodative component and near-distance disparity.
   (d) Objective measurement tests are superior to subjective tests in determining the deviation that should be corrected.

Answer: (a) Prism adaptation test should be performed even in absence of binocularity as these patients often demonstrate binocular functions after ocular alignment. Angle measured by objective tests should be the target angle for correction.

2. *Incorrect* statement regarding lost/slipped/severed/PITS muscle?
   (a) Partial thickness suture placement through the muscle can lead to these complications.
   (b) Muscle that is too tight or fibrosed may get torn at the muscle-tendon junction resulting in 'pulled-in-two syndrome' (PITS).
   (c) The globe can be slightly enophthalmic and the palpebral fissure decreased as patients attempt to move the eye in the direction of the lost muscle.

(d) Imaging is helpful in localization of the muscle as well as identifying absence or presence of its attachments to the globe.

Answer: (c) The globe can be slightly proptotic and the palpebral fissure widened with limitation of movement in the direction of action of lost muscle.

3. *False* statement regarding strabismus surgery?
    (a) Late-onset consecutive strabismus occurs due to remodelling of scar tissue.
    (b) Scleral perforation and penetration usually occur during muscle disinsertion or muscle reattachment.
    (c) Risk of perforation is higher in recession than in other strabismus procedure.
    (d) Recession results in dellen formation more frequently than resection.

Answer: (d) Resection results in more frequent dellen formation, as resection involves more tissue crowding near limbus than recession.

4. Which of the following statement is *correct* regarding anterior segment ischaemia following strabismus surgery?
    (a) Fornix incisions have a lower incidence compared to limbal incisions.
    (b) Vessel sparing surgery does not reduce its risk.
    (c) Its incidence is irrespective of type of procedure.
    (d) It is more commonly seen in young patients.

Answer: (a) Fornix incisions spare anterior ciliary vessels reducing its incidence. Vessel sparing surgery reduces the risk but does not eliminate it. It is commoner in multiple muscle surgeries and transposition procedures. It is commoner in elderly and debilitated patients.

5. Causes of overcorrection/undercorrection are all *except*?
    (a) Lateral gaze incomitance
    (b) Amblyopia
    (c) Eccentric fixation
    (d) Good binocularity

Answer: (d) Good binocularity reduces the unsatisfactory motor outcome. All other options listed above increase it.

References

1. Shen E, Porco T, Rutar T. Errors in strabismus surgery. JAMA Ophthalmol. 2013;131(1):75–9.
2. MacEwen C, Gregson R. Complications of strabismus surgery – how to avoid and manage them. In: Manual of strabismus surgery. UK: Butterworth-Heinemann; 2003. p. 172–3.
3. Parks MM. Slipped, disinserted or severed and lost muscles. In: Clinical strabismus management. Philadelphia: W. B. Saunders; 1999. p. 529–38.

4. Plager DA, Parks MM. Recognition and repair of slipped rectus muscle. J Pediatr Ophthalmol Strabismus. 1988;25:270–4.
5. Parks MM, Bloom JN. The "slipped" muscle. Ophthalmology. 1979;86:1389–96.
6. Wallace DK, Steven RV, Mukherji SK. Strabismus surgery complicated by "pulled-in-two syndrome" in a case of breast carcinoma metastatic to the medial rectus muscle. J AAPOS. 2000;4:117–9.
7. Dunbar JA, Lueder GT. Intraoperative dehiscence of a rectus muscle: report of two cases. J AAPOS. 1997;1:175–7.
8. Kowal L, Wutthiphan S, McKelvie P. The snapped inferior rectus. Aust N Z Ophthalmol. 1998;26:29–35.
9. Chatzistefanou KI, Kushner BJ, Gentry LR. Magnetic resonance imaging of the arc of contact of extraocular muscles: implications regarding the incidence of slipped muscles. J AAPOS. 2000;4(2):84–93.
10. Sebastian RT, Marsh IB. Adjustment of the surgical nomogram for surgery on slipped EOMs. J AAPOS. 2006;10:573–6.
11. Demer JL, Oh SY, Poukens V. Evidence for active control of rectus extraocular muscle pulleys. Invest Ophthalmol Vis Sci. 2000;41(6):1280–90.
12. Awad AH, Mullaney PB, Al-Hazmi A, et al. Recognized globe perforation during strabismus surgery: incidence, risk factors, and sequelae. J AAPOS. 2000;4(3):150 153.
13. Fresina M, Campos EC. Corneal "dellen" as a complication of strabismus surgery. Eye (Lond). 2009;23(1):161–3.
14. Guadilla AM, de Liaño PG, Merino P, Franco G. Conjunctival cysts as a complication after strabismus surgery. J Pediatr Ophthalmol Strabismus. 2011;48(5):298–300.
15. Khan AO, Al-Katan H, Al-Baharna I, Al-Wadani F. Infected epithelial inclusion cyst mimicking subconjunctival abscess after strabismus surgery. J AAPOS. 2007;11(3):303–4.
16. Kushner BJ. Subconjunctival cysts as a complication of strabismus surgery. Arch Ophthalmol. 1992;110(9):1243–5.
17. Murray AD. Slipped and lost muscles and other tales of the unexpected: Phillip Knapp Lecture. J AAPOS. 1998;2:133–43.
18. Ginat D, Sadiq MA, Dagi LR. Imaging of strabismus and craniofacial malformation surgery. In: Ginat D, Freitag S, editors. Post-treatment imaging of the orbit. NY: Springer; 2014. p. 132–3.
19. Waite C, Dai S. Orbital imaging to identify a "lost" lateral rectus muscle. J Pediatr Ophthalmol Strabismus. 2016;53:e32–4.
20. von Noorden GK, Campos EC. Chapter 16: Esodeviations. In: Binocular vision and ocular motility. 6th ed. St. Louis: Mosby; 2002. p. 311–49.
21. von Noorden GK, Campos EC. Chapter 17: Exodeviations. In: Binocular vision and ocular motility. 6th ed. St. Louis: Mosby; 2002. p. 356–76.
22. Kraft SP. Selected exotropia entities and principles of management. In: Rosenbaum AL, Santiago AP, editors. Clinical strabismus management. Philadelphia: W. B. Saunders; 1999. p. 193–9.
23. Noh JE, Park KH, Lee J, Jung MS, Kim SY. Changes in refractive error and anterior segment parameters after isolated lateral rectus muscle recession. J AAPOS. 2013;17:291–5.
24. Al-Tamimi E, Al-Nosair G, Yassin S. Effect of horizontal strabismus surgery on the refractive status. Strabismus. 2015;23(3):111–6.
25. Dottan SA, Hoffman P, Oliver MD. Astigmatism after strabismus surgery. Ophthalmic Surg Las. 1988;19:128–9.
26. von Noorden GK, Campos EC. Principles of surgical treatment. In: Binocular vision and ocular motility: theory and management of strabismus. 6th ed. St. Louis, MO: CV Mosby; 2001. p. 571–3.
27. Santos de Souza Lima LC, Velarde LG, Vianna RN, Herzog Neto G. The effect of horizontal strabismus surgery on the vertical palpebral fissure width. J AAPOS. 2011;15(5):473–5.
28. Lagrèze WA, Gerling J, Staubach F. Changes of the lid fissure after surgery on horizontal extraocular muscles. Am J Ophthalmol. 2005;140(6):1145–6.

29. Akbari MR, Raygan F, Ameri A, Jafari A, Eshraghi B, Fard MA. Lower eyelid retractor lysis versus Lockwood advancement to minimize lower eyelid retraction resulting from inferior rectus muscle recession. J AAPOS. 2013;17(4):445–7.
30. Simon JW, Lininger LL, Scheraga JL. Recognized sclera perforation during eye muscle surgery: incidence and sequelae. J Pediatr Ophthalmol Strabismus. 1992;29(5):273–5.
31. Bleik JH, Cherfan GM. Anterior segment ischemia after the Jensen procedure in a 10-year-old patient. Am J Ophthalmol. 1995;119(4):524–5.
32. Wolf E, Wagner RS, Zarbin MA. Anterior segment ischemia and retinal detachment after vertical rectus muscle surgery. Eur J Ophthalmol. 2000;10(1):82–7.
33. Saunders RA, Phillips MS. Anterior segment ischemia after three rectus muscle surgery. Ophthalmology. 1988;95(4):533–7.
34. Murdock TJ, Mills MD. Anterior segment ischemia after strabismus surgery with microvascular dissection. J AAPOS. 2000;4(1):56–7.
35. von Noorden GK, Campos EC. Principles of surgical treatment. In: von Noorden GK, Campos EC, editors. Binocular vision and ocular motility. 6th ed. St. Louis: Mosby; 2002. p. 620–1.

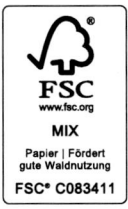